Legg-Calvé-Perthes Disease

Guest Editors

CHARLES T. PRICE, MD
BENJAMIN JOSEPH, MS Orth, MCh Orth

ORTHOPEDIC CLINICS OF NORTH AMERICA

www.orthopedic.theclinics.com

July 2011 • Volume 42 • Number 3

SAUNDERS an imprint of ELSEVIER, Inc.

W.B. SAUNDERS COMPANY
A Division of Elsevier Inc.

1600 John F. Kennedy Blvd. • Suite 1800 • Philadelphia, PA 19103-2899.

http://www.orthopedic.theclinics.com

ORTHOPEDIC CLINICS OF NORTH AMERICA Volume 42, Number 3
July 2011 ISSN 0030-5898, ISBN-13: 978-1-4557-1046-1

Editor: Debora Dellapena

Photocopying

Single photocopies of single articles may be made for personal use as allowed by national copyright laws. Permission of the Publisher and payment of a fee is required for all other photocopying, including multiple or systematic copying, copying for advertising or promotional purposes, resale, and all forms of document delivery. Special rates are available for educational institutions that wish to make photocopies for non-profit educational classroom use. For information on how to seek permission visit www.elsevier.com/permissions or call: (+44) 1865 843830 (UK)/(+1) 215 239 3804 (USA).

Derivative Works

Subscribers may reproduce tables of contents or prepare lists of articles including abstracts for internal circulation within their institutions. Permission of the Publisher is required for resale or distribution outside the institution. Permission of the Publisher is required for all other derivative works, including compilations and translations (please consult www.elsevier.com/permissions).

Electronic Storage or Usage

Permission of the Publisher is required to store or use electronically any material contained in this journal, including any article or part of an article (please consult www.elsevier.com/permissions). Except as outlined above, no part of this publication may be reproduced, stored in a retrieval system or transmitted in any form or by any means, electronic, mechanical, photocopying, recording or otherwise, without prior written permission of the Publisher.

Notice

No responsibility is assumed by the Publisher for any injury and/or damage to persons or property as a matter of products liability, negligence or otherwise, or from any use or operation of any methods, products, instructions or ideas contained in the material herein. Because of rapid advances in the medical sciences, in particular, independent verification of diagnoses and drug dosages should be made.

Although all advertising material is expected to conform to ethical (medical) standards, inclusion in this publication does not constitute a guarantee or endorsement of the quality or value of such product or of the claims made of it by its manufacturer.

Orthopedic Clinics of North America (ISSN 0030-5898) is published quarterly by Elsevier Inc., 360 Park Avenue South, New York, NY 10010-1710. Months of issue are January, April, July, and October. Business and Editorial Offices: 1600 John F. Kennedy Blvd., Suite 1800, Philadelphia, PA 19103-2899. Customer Service Office: 3251 Riverport Lane, Maryland Heights, MO 63043. Periodicals postage paid at New York, NY and additional mailing offices. Subscription prices are $269.00 per year for (US individuals), $513.00 per year for (US institutions), $318.00 per year (Canadian individuals), $615.00 per year (Canadian institutions), $392.00 per year (international individuals), $615.00 per year (international institutions), $132.00 per year (US students), $191.00 per year (Canadian and international students). Foreign air speed delivery is included in all *Clinics* subscription prices. All prices are subject to change without notice. **POSTMASTER:** Send change of address to *Orthopedic Clinics of North America*, **Elsevier Health Sciences Division, Subscription Customer Service, 3251 Riverport Lane, Maryland Heights, MO 63043. Customer Service (orders, claims, online, change of address): Elsevier Health Sciences Division, Subscription Customer Service, 3251 Riverport Lane, Maryland Heights, MO 63043. Tel: 1-800-654-2452 (U.S. and Canada); 314-447-8871 (outside U.S. and Canada). Fax: 314-447-8029. E-mail: journalscustomerservice-usa@elsevier. com (for print support); journalsonlinesupport-usa@elsevier.com (for online support).**

Reprints. For copies of 100 or more, of articles in this publication, please contact the Commercial Reprints Department, Elsevier Inc., 360 Park Avenue South, New York, NY 10010-1710. Tel.: 212-633-3812; Fax: 212-462-1935; E-mail: reprints@elsevier. com.

Orthopedic Clinics of North America is covered in *MEDLINE/PubMed* (*Index Medicus*), *Cinahl, Excerpta Medica,* and *Cumulative Index to Nursing and Allied Health Literature.*

Printed and bound by CPI Group (UK) Ltd, Croydon, CR0 4YY
Transferred to Digital Print 2011

Contributors

GUEST EDITORS

CHARLES T. PRICE, MD
Director, Pediatric Orthopaedic Education;
Associate Director, Orthopaedic Residency
Program, Arnold Palmer Hospital for Children;
Professor of Orthopedic Surgery, University
of Central Florida College of Medicine,
Orlando, Florida

BENJAMIN JOSEPH, MS Orth, MCh Orth
Professor of Orthopaedics and Head
of Paediatric Orthopaedic Service,
Paediatric Orthopaedic Service, Kasturba
Medical College, Manipal,
Karnataka State, India

AUTHORS

FEDERICO CANAVESE, MD, PhD
Service de Chirurgie Infantile, Centre
Hospitalier Universitaire Estaing, Clermont
Ferrand, France

TAE-JOON CHO, MD
Division of Pediatric Orthopaedics, Seoul
National University Children's Hospital,
Seoul, Korea

IN HO CHOI, MD
Professor, Division of Pediatric Orthopaedics,
Seoul National University Children's Hospital,
Seoul, Korea

JOHN CLOHISY, MD
Department of Orthopaedic Surgery,
Washington University School of Medicine,
St Louis, Missouri

CHRISTOPHER R. COSTA, MD
Research Fellow, Center for Joint Preservation
and Replacement, Rubin Institute for
Advanced Orthopedics, Sinai Hospital of
Baltimore, Baltimore, Maryland

ANTOINE DE GHELDERE, MD
Consultant Paediatric Orthopaedic Surgeon,
Department of Orthopaedics, The Great North
Children's Hospital, Newcastle Upon Tyne,
United Kingdom

ALAIN DIMEGLIO, MD
Université de Montpellier, Faculté de
Médecine, Montpellier, France

DEBORAH M. EASTWOOD, FRCS
Consultant Paediatric Orthopaedic Surgeon,
The Catterall Unit, The Royal National
Orthopaedic Hospital, Stanmore, Middlesex,
United Kingdom

**ANDREW J. HALL, MB BS, MSc, PhD,
FRCP, FFPH, FMedSci**
Professor of Epidemiology, Department
of Infectious Disease Epidemiology, London
School of Hygiene and Tropical Medicine,
London, United Kingdom

JOSÉ A. HERRERA-SOTO, MD
Director, Pediatric Orthopedics, Arnold
Palmer Hospital for Children,
Orlando, Florida

JOHN A. HERRING, MD
Professor, Department of Orthopaedic
Surgery, University of Texas Southwestern
Medical Center; Chief of Staff, Texas Scottish
Rite Hospital for Children, Dallas, Texas

HARISH S. HOSALKAR, MD
Department of Orthopaedic Surgery, Rady
Children's Hospital San Diego, University
of California, San Diego,
San Diego, California

GAMAL AHMED HOSNY, MD
Professor of Orthopaedic Surgery,
Department of Orthopaedics, Benha
Faculty of Medicine, Benha University,
Maadi, Cairo, Egypt

AARON J. JOHNSON, MD
Research Fellow, Center for Joint
Preservation and Replacement, Rubin Institute
for Advanced Orthopedics, Sinai Hospital
of Baltimore, Baltimore, Maryland

BENJAMIN JOSEPH, MS Orth, MCh Orth
Professor of Orthopaedics and Head of
Paediatric Orthopaedic Service, Paediatric
Orthopaedic Service, Kasturba Medical
College, Manipal, Karnataka State, India

HARRY K.W. KIM, MD, MSc, FRCSC
Director of Research, Center for Excellence
in Hip Disorders, Research Department, Texas
Scottish Rite Hospital for Children; Associate
Professor, Department of Orthopaedic
Surgery, University of Texas Southwestern
Medical Center, Dallas, Texas

YOUNG-JO KIM, MD, PhD
Department of Orthopaedic Surgery,
Children's Hospital Boston, Boston,
Massachusetts

DAVID G. LITTLE, MBBS, FRACS(Orth), PhD
Senior Staff Specialist and Head, Orthopaedic
Research; Department of Orthopaedics, The
Children's Hospital at Westmead, Westmead;
Professor, Discipline of Paediatrics and Child
Health, University of Sydney, Sydney,
New South Wales, Australia

MICHAEL A. MONT, MD
Director, Center for Joint Preservation and
Replacement, Rubin Institute for Advanced
Orthopedics, Sinai Hospital of Baltimore,
Baltimore, Maryland

HYUK JU MOON, MD
Division of Pediatric Orthopaedics,
Seoul National University Children's Hospital,
Seoul, Korea

QAIS NAZIRI, MD
Research Fellow, Center for Joint
Preservation and Replacement, Rubin Institute
for Advanced Orthopedics, Sinai Hospital
of Baltimore, Baltimore, Maryland

EDUARDO N. NOVAIS, MD
Department of Orthopaedic Surgery,
Children's Hospital-Boston, Boston,
Massachusetts

DROR PALEY, MD, FRCSC
Paley Advanced Limb Lengthening Institute,
West Palm Beach, Florida

**DANIEL C. PERRY, MB ChB(Hons),
MRCS (Eng)**
Monk Research Fellow, Department of Child
Health, University of Liverpool, Liverpool,
United Kingdom

DAVID PODESZWA, MD
Texas Scottish Rite Hospital, Dallas, Texas

CHARLES T. PRICE, MD
Director, Pediatric Orthopaedic Education;
Associate Director, Orthopaedic Residency
Program, Arnold Palmer Hospital for Children;
Professor of Orthopedic Surgery, University
of Central Florida College of Medicine,
Orlando, Florida

KENT A. REINKER, MD
Clinical Professor of Orthopaedics,
University of Texas Health Science Center,
San Antonio, Texas

KLAUS SIEBENROCK, MD
Department of Orthopaedic Surgery,
University of Bern, Bern, Switzerland

SHAWN C. STANDARD, MD
Head of Pediatric Orthopedics, International
Center for Limb Lengthening, Rubin Institute
for Advanced Orthopedics, Sinai Hospital
of Baltimore, Baltimore, Maryland

DANIEL SUCATO, MD
Texas Scottish Rite Hospital, Dallas, Texas

GEORGE H. THOMPSON, MD
Director of Pediatric Orthopaedics,
Rainbow Babies and Children Hospital;
Professor, Orthopaedic Surgery and
Pediatrics Case Western Reserve University,
Cleveland, Ohio

DENNIS R. WENGER, MD
Clinical Professor, Department of
Orthopaedic Surgery, Rady Children's
Hospital San Diego, University of California,
San Diego, San Diego, California

WON JOON YOO, MD
Division of Pediatric Orthopaedics,
Seoul National University Children's Hospital,
Seoul, Korea

Contents

SECTION I–THE DISEASE

> The incidence of Perthes disease varies markedly both between countries and within countries down to a local level. The disease is more common in white than in Asian or black African children. The disease is associated with deprivation; with a steep disease gradient across social class groups. This epidemiology alongside the lack of concordance in twins suggests a strong environmental etiology, with little evidence to suggest a genetic predisposition. Children are frequently short, with a growth pattern described as "rostral-sparing". A propensity to associated congenital anomalies suggests an intrauterine cause.

> Since the original reports of Legg-Calvé-Perthes disease (LCPD), much research effort has been undertaken to improve understanding of this idiopathic hip disorder. This article focuses on the current knowledge of the pathophysiology, classifications, and natural history of LCPD. Although the cause of LCPD remains largely unknown, some insight has been gained on its pathophysiology through experimental studies using animal models of ischemic necrosis. The few available clinical studies on the natural history of LCPD suggest that femoral head deformity is well tolerated in short and intermediate terms, but 50% of patients develop disabling arthritis in the sixth decade of life.

> Imaging in Legg-Calvé-Perthes disease should help assess the severity and the stage of the disease, detect severe forms earlier, and provide guidance to therapy. However, due to the complexity of the disease, not all examinations can be performed at the same time with the same goals. The scope of this work is to provide an overview of all imaging techniques available today, and to help understand when to use a particular examination. Advantages and limitations of plain radiographs, bone scintigraphy, magnetic resonance imaging, arthrography, computed tomography, and ultrasonography are identified.

> The shape of the femoral head at the time when Perthes disease heals is the most important determinant of the risk for degenerative arthritis; hence, the shape of the femoral head and congruence of the hip are the most useful outcome measures. Although several prognostic factors that predict femoral head deformation may be identified during the course of Perthes disease, only two prognostic factors may be identified early enough to institute preventive intervention: femoral head extrusion

and the age at onset of the disease. Femoral head extrusion is the only factor that may be influenced by treatment.

of hinge abduction allows the lateral acetabular ossification center to grow more normally.

Shelf and/or Reduction and Containment Surgery   355

Kent A. Reinker

Hinge abduction occurs early in the fragmentation stage of Legg-Calvé-Perthes disease and should be suspected when abduction and internal rotation are lost. It can be confirmed by an AP radiograph in abduction and internal rotation in which the ossific nucleus is not covered by the acetabulum. An arthrogram can then yield greater information regarding the reversibility of the hinge abduction. Hinge abduction should be considered a contraindication to containment by redirectional pelvic or femoral varus osteotomy. However, good results have been reported with acetabular augmentation via shelf procedures or Chiari osteotomies. Valgus femoral osteotomies have also been beneficial in the treatment of the Legg-Calvé-Perthes hip with hinge abduction.

Articulated Distraction   361

Gamal Ahmed Hosny

Articular hip distraction can be applied either by using a monolateral articulated distractor or a circular fixator. The fixator should be aligned such that its axis is aligned with the transverse axis of the hip joint. Following distraction, the range of motion is maintained with regular physiotherapy. It is a useful salvage procedure in older children with hip stiffness, when other methods of containment are not applicable.

SECTION IV–TREATMENT AFTER COMPLETE HEALING OF PERTHES' DISEASE

Principles of Treating the Sequelae of Perthes Disease   365

Dennis R. Wenger and Harish S. Hosalkar

Despite early treatment efforts, many patients with Perthes disease are left with residual femoral head deformity, which can be symptomatic with a residual limp and poor hip motion. Many such patients can be treated using an extra-articular femoral osteotomy. Selecting treatment methods for patients with symptomatic Perthes disease with healed but deformed femoral heads has always been difficult but is now even more complex because of the new possibilities of femoral head–neck recontouring and femoral head reduction surgery. Occasionally, patients develop osteochondritis dissecans when there is little femoral head deformity. The primary objective of management is to establish the exact cause of pain and address that cause specifically. This article outlines an approach to these patients.

Treatment of Coxa Brevis   373

Shawn C. Standard

Coxa brevis of the hip results in a morphologic change of the proximal femur creating pain and fatigue, leg-length discrepancy, and altered gait. The most common cause is a growth alteration of the proximal femoral physis secondary to ischemic necrosis of the proximal femoral epiphysis. This article describes the Morscher osteotomy—a unique femoral neck-lengthening technique. The outcomes of this successful and predictable technique are resolution of symptoms of fatigue and hip discomfort; the absence of nonunion, infection, or hardware failure; and restoration of normal proximal femoral morphology and biomechanics.

The aspherical coxa magna femoral head can be made more spherical by intra-articular osteotomy. The Ganz technique of femoral head reduction osteotomy to reduce the size and restore the spherical shape of the femoral head has been performed in 20 patients over the past 5 years. A good or excellent functional and radiographic result was obtained in 14 of the 20. A fair result (decreased pain but no improvement in range of motion) occurred in 3, and a poor result (stiffness and pain) occurred in 3. The preliminary results of this technique are therefore very promising.

Healed Legg-Calvé-Perthes disease may cause both intra-articular and extra-articular impingement, resulting in a symptomatic hip prior to the onset of osteoarthritis. Various impingement-relieving surgeries have been used in the past; however, the development of the safe surgical dislocation technique has allowed a better understanding of complex deformity that may be present in these hips and hence may improve treatment of these symptomatic prearthritic hips. This article outlines the range of deformities possible in a Perthes hip, and treatment strategies to surgically address these deformities. For Perthes disease good preoperative clinical and radiographic assessment is essential, and intraoperative assessment vital.

Patients with Legg-Calvé-Perthes disease can often be successfully treated with femoral head–preserving measures, such as bracing, or containment procedures with osteotomies. However, in some cases, after resolution of the disease, the femoral head may proceed to collapse or progress to severe arthritis at a young age. If nonoperative methods have failed, the only treatment options available for these adolescents or young adults may be a total hip resurfacing or a total hip arthroplasty (THA). This article focuses on the results and unique technical considerations of resurfacing and THA for patients who have severe hip osteoarthritis after resolved Legg-Calvé-Perthes disease.

SECTION V–NEWER TREATMENT OPTIONS

Standard surgical approaches for Perthes disease consist of nonoperative physical treatments or surgical treatment. Several investigators have been working on a better understanding of the pathophysiology and pathobiology of Perthes disease. Most of the focus has been on antiresorptive treatments. Other treatment avenues, however, include controlling the inflammatory phase of Perthes disease, increasing revascularization of necrotic bone, and anabolic strategies to increase bone formation. This article presents a current pathophysiological model of Perthes disease, reviews experimental strategies in pharmaceutical treatments, and suggests future areas for research.

Core decompression may be used as adjunct for treatment in some cases of Legg-Calvé-Perthes disease (LCPD). The primary application is for patients with onset at 12 years of age or older. We recommend classifying these older patients as idiopathic juvenile osteonecrosis and treating them similarly to adults with avascular necrosis. Juvenile osteonecrosis may benefit from core decompression combined with shelf acetabuloplasty during the early stages of necrosis. Younger children with LCPD may benefit from decompression by fenestration of the femoral head. Experience in adult-onset osteonecrosis and our early experience suggest that some patients may benefit from these adjunctive treatments.

Orthopedic Clinics of North America

THE CLINICS ARE NOW AVAILABLE ONLINE!

Access your subscription at:
www.theclinics.com

Preface
Legg-Calvé-Perthes Disease

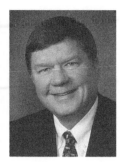
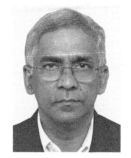

Charles T. Price, MD   Benjamin Joseph, MS Orth, MCh Orth

Guest Editors

A hundred years after the description of Legg-Calvé-Perthes disease, the aetiology remains elusive and a great deal of confusion abounds regarding issues related to the treatment of this enigmatic disease. It is against this unenviable background that we set out to put together this symposium on Legg-Calvé-Perthes disease.

The symposium has been divided into five sections; in the first section Hall and Perry review the current state of our knowledge (or the lack of it) of the aetiology of Legg-Calvé-Perthes disease and elegantly summarize the fascinating epidemiological aspects of the disease. They conclude quite appropriately that there is a dire need for more well-designed epidemiological studies if we are to unravel the mystery of the underlying cause of the disease. The reviews of Kim, Herring, and Dimeglio put into perspective our knowledge of the pathogenesis of the disease and the role of imaging in monitoring the disease and planning treatment. Joseph critically analyses the value of prognostic factors in planning treatment.

The three subsequent sections are devoted to treatment of the disease. Ideally, treatment of Legg-Calvé-Perthes disease should aim to prevent femoral head deformation and this is only possible if intervention is instituted before the head begins to deform. Joseph and Price outline the principles of such early preventive intervention. Price, Thompson, and Wenger discuss various options for early containment. Once treatment is delayed, the aim of treatment shifts from preventing deformity to minimizing deformity and dealing with complications such as hinge abduction. Choi lays down the principles of treatment at this stage, while Eastwood, Reinker, and Hosny describe the treatment modalities. The treatment of established femoral head deformity and arthritis following Legg-Calvé-Perthes disease require totally different strategies and Wenger and Hosalker discuss the principles. Standard, Paley, Kim, and Mont describe elaborate and innovative ways of salvaging these hips.

In the last section, newer methods of treatment that have shown promise in experimental animal models are discussed by Little, Kim, and Herrera-Soto.

One of our aims was to try to clarify areas of confusion related to treatment recommendations that have appeared in the literature. It was our hope that some semblance of agreement could be reached among the contributors to this symposium regarding the basic principles of treatment of Legg-Calvé-Perthes disease.

Based on the articles in this issue, we put together a consensus statement which we circulated among the contributors and this we include in the end of the symposium. We were encouraged to note that there is a great deal more agreement than what one is lead to believe.

Charles T. Price, MD
Arnold Palmer Hospital for Children
Pediatric Orthopaedic Division
83 West Columbia Street
Orlando, FL 32806, USA

Benjamin Joseph, MS Orth, MCh Orth
Paediatric Orthopaedic Service
Kasturba Medical College
Manipal 576 104
Karnataka State, India

E-mail addresses:
charles.price@orlandohealth.com (C.T. Price)
bjosephortho@yahoo.co.in (B. Joseph)

Orthop Clin N Am 42 (2011) xi
doi:10.1016/j.ocl.2011.04.011

The Epidemiology and Etiology of Perthes Disease

Daniel C. Perry, MB ChB(Hons), MRCS (Eng)[a],*,
Andrew J. Hall, MB BS, MSc, PhD, FRCP, FFPH, FMedSci[b]

KEYWORDS

• Epidemiology • Etiology • Perthes • Geography • Incidence

Perthes disease occurs in around 5 boys for every affected girl. The disease affects children between 2 and 14 years old with the peak age of onset, among white children, being 5 years old. The age of onset has been demonstrated to be later among Indian children.[1] Approximately 15% of cases are bilateral.

GEOGRAPHY

There is a marked geographic variation in the frequency of Perthes disease. Studies of incidence are difficult to directly compare, as inappropriate population denominators have sometimes been used. **Table 1** shows those studies where the annual incidence rates have been calculated using a denominator of 0- to 14-year-old child years.

There is a significant geographic variation in disease incidence between countries, within countries, and even between small local areas. Equatorial regions have a low incidence of disease while Northern Europe has the highest documented incidence. This divergence may at least partly be explained by race, because evidence from the Eastern Cape of South Africa shows that black African children living alongside African whites have a substantially lower disease incidence, and people of mixed race an intermediate level (black: 0.45; mixed race: 1.7; white: 10.8 per 100,000 children 0–14 years old).[5] Investigators from predominantly white countries, with significant black populations, have similarly identified few cases of Perthes disease among black children, New York, USA: 14 black children among 358 Perthes disease cases[15]; Connecticut, USA: 2 black children among 203 cases[19]; Massachusetts, USA: 1 black child amongst 86 cases.[2] Population studies from Asian countries have found an incidence between that of black and white individuals, with incidence rates of 0.93 per 100,000 children 0 to 14 years old from a population study of Japan,[13] and 3.85 per 100,000 children 0 to 14 years old in Korea (see **Table 1**).[11]

There is data to show regional disease distributions within three countries, namely England, India, and Norway. All show a variation in incidence of at least twofold. In England the southern region of Wessex had half the incidence of Merseyside in the North West, with Trent in the Midlands having an intermediate value (11.1 vs 7.6 vs 5.5 cases per 100,000 children 0–14 years old per annum).[4] In India, incidence in Vellore (south-east) was 0.4 per 100,000 per annum for 0- to 14-year-olds whereas in Manipal (south-west) it was 4.4.[1] In Norway, an incidence of 3.6 in Northern Finmark county contrasted with 16.7 per 100,000 per annum in Western Sogn og Fjordane.[14]

Incidence even varies notably within small areas. This divergence was first demonstrated within Merseyside (United Kingdom), with a very high incidence in inner-city Liverpool prompting investigators to examine the relationship between deprivation and disease.[6,10] A steep social class gradient of disease from 4 per 100,000 per annum

The authors have nothing to disclose.
a Department of Child Health, University of Liverpool, Liverpool, L12 2AP, UK
b Department of Infectious Disease Epidemiology, London School of Hygiene and Tropical Medicine, Keppel Street, London, WC1E 7HT, UK
* Corresponding author.
E-mail address: danperry@doctors.org.uk

Orthop Clin N Am 42 (2011) 279–283
doi:10.1016/j.ocl.2011.03.002

Table 1
Annual incidence of Perthes disease in children aged 0 to 14 years by country and region

Year	Study	Location	Annual Incidence Figures per 100,000 Population (0–14 y old)		
			Males	Females	Overall
1966	Molloy and MacMahon[2]	Massachusetts, USA	—	—	5.7
1972	Gray et al[3]	British Columbia, Canada	8.4	1.6	5.1
1978	Barker et al[4]	Wessex, UK	8.7	2.0	5.5
1978	Barker et al[4]	Merseyside, UK	16.9	5.0	11.1
1978	Barker et al[4]	Trent, UK	12.0	3.0	7.6
1982	Purry[5]	Eastern Cape, South Africa (Blacks)	—	—	0.5
1982	Purry[5]	Eastern Cape, South Africa (Mixed race)	—	—	1.7
1982	Purry[5]	Eastern Cape, South Africa (Whites)	—	—	10.8
1983	Hall et al[6]	Liverpool, UK	25.8	4.9	15.6
1988	Joseph et al[1]	Vellore, Eastern India	—	—	0.4
1988	Joseph et al[1]	Udupi, Western India	—	—	4.4
1989	Hall and Barker[7]	Yorkshire, UK	—	—	6.1
1992	Moberg and Rehnberg[8]	Uppsala, Sweden	8.5	2.1	6.3
2000	Kealey et al[9]	Northern Ireland	—	—	11.6
2001	Margetts et al[10]	Liverpool, UK	—	—	8.7
2005	Rowe et al[11]	Korea	6.1	1.5	3.8
2005	Pillai et al[12]	Southwest Scotland	—	—	15.4
2006	Kim et al[13]	Japan	1.5	0.2	0.9
2006	Wiig et al[14]	Norway	—	—	9.2

in Social Class 1 (highest social standing) to 31.7 per 100,000 per annum in Social Class 5 (lowest social standing) was found.[6] Similar social class and deprivation trends have now been reported by several other studies,[12,16] although this association is not universally demonstrated.[17]

TIME TRENDS

Few studies have sought to measure the influence of time on disease incidence. Between 1924 and 1960, Peic[18] reviewed outpatient data from an orthopedic clinic in Dortmund, Germany. He noted that the incidence of cases tended to increase 5 years after a period of economic recession. However, his method of case ascertainment and definition of source population raises doubts as to the robustness of this association. A Scottish study similarly noted an association between "gross value added" (a measure of regional wealth) and the incidence of Perthes disease, though the period of observation was just 10 years and case numbers were small.[12] The only area to record trends in disease incidence over a prolonged period is Merseyside.[6,10] The disease incidence has been measured from 1976, with the last

published data considering the period up to 1995. The incidence within Liverpool was found to have halved between the 1976 and 1995, with rates falling from 16.9 to 8.7 cases per 100,000 per annum. This time period was associated with a progressive increase in the standard of living within the city, which may account for the decline in incidence.

The pattern of variation in incidence by social class, over small geographic areas, and with time all indicate a major environmental influence in the cause of the disease. This influence appears to act early in childhood or in prenatal life. Family studies show that in large case series disease occurs in approximately 0.5% to 0.8% of the parents and 2% to 4% of siblings of affected children.[3,19,20] Twin pairs within such case series have identified 10 dizygous pairs and 5 monozygous pairs, each with a single concordant pair.[19,21–23] Given this low concordance in twins, it seems likely that familial aggregation is attributable to a shared environment rather than a genetic susceptibility.

Analysis of the age distribution of onset of cases shows that it conforms to a log-normal distribution.[24] This pattern is typical of incubation periods and is consistent with a single exposure acting at a critical period in the hip development, either prenatally or in the first 2 years of life.

ASSOCIATIONS
Stature

The most detailed observation of growth in Perthes disease was published in 1978.[25] This large, cross-sectional, anthropometric study involved 232 children with Perthes disease from 3 centers in the United Kingdom. A control group was drawn from primary schools in 2 of the 3 regions. The results demonstrated a subtle global growth disturbance in affected individuals with the demonstration of a normal head size, yet increasing growth restriction as one progressed distally along limb units, such that the hands and feet were most disproportionate compared with head size: a pattern of dysmorphism described as "rostral sparing" (**Fig. 1**). Given the strong socioeconomic gradient of Perthes disease, it was however unclear whether this growth abnormality was a function of urban deprivation or a true disease-related phenomenon. A further study therefore sought to compare anthropometry in siblings of affected children matching for urban deprivation as well as other familial factors.[26] This study of 38 cases and 49 sibling controls demonstrated a clear growth restriction most notable in the feet of affected children (see **Fig. 1**).

This association with abnormal growth and the possibility of an intrauterine cause raises the question of whether there is an association with shape and size at birth of the affected children.

Birth Proportions

Birth weight has been studied in several settings, but no association with Perthes disease has been consistently found.[14,23,27] The study of birth weight is problematic given the potential confounding variables including socioeconomic status, parity, and parental smoking. Thus a recent Swedish study by Bahmanyar and colleagues[28] considered smoking, gestational age, and birth weight simultaneously, concluding that an association exists between birth weight of less than 1500 g and Perthes disease (odds ratio [OR] 3.46, 95% confidence interval [CI] 1.11–10.84). The wide confidence intervals indicate the small number of cases falling within this group (9 of 731 cases). It is possible that this association resulted from avascular necrosis precipitated by steroid use for neonatal chronic lung disease rather than true Perthes disease.

A Norwegian birth registry study is the first to show an association with birth length.[14] The risk of Perthes disease was increased by 50% in those under 50 cm at birth compared with those over 50 cm. Although little account of confounding was made, in particular of socioeconomic status, this is the first study to examine, and find, that the growth abnormality was present at birth.

Congenital Malformations

One influence of an intrauterine exposure might be on congenital malformations. Catterall and colleagues[29] originally demonstrated an association between Perthes disease and inguinal hernias and genitourinary malformations, with the frequency of an inguinal hernia being 8 times the expected number. Other series have failed to replicate genitourinary associations,[19,21] but recently the association with undescended testicles was found using the Medical Birth Registry of Norway.[14] Other associations such as inguinal hernias could not be examined, as such details are not recorded in this birth register, but a strong association with Down syndrome was found. A case-control study in Nottingham (United Kingdom) of minor congenital abnormalities using standardized criteria and a single observer found a marked increase in Perthes-affected children, with nearly half exhibiting one of the abnormalities versus 23% of controls.[30]

HYPOTHESES

The clear association with growth and the potential for an intrauterine effect have led to two specific hypotheses: nutritional deficiency and parental smoking.

Manganese deficiency has so far been investigated because of the known consequences of growth abnormalities in chickens, and epiphyseal dysplasia in rats. An initial case-control study amongst children with Perthes disease found an association,[31] but this was not confirmed in a

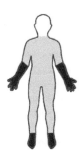

Normal (White)
- *Head – Normal Size*

Restricted Growth (Grey)
- *Sitting Height – Reduced*

Most Significant Growth Restriction (Black)
- *Hands and forearms small relative to upper arm*
- *Feet small relative to tibia*

Fig. 1. Pattern of abnormal growth in Perthes disease. (*Modified from* Burwell R, Dangerfield P, Hall D, et al. Perthes' disease. An anthropometric study revealing impaired and disproportionate growth. J Bone Joint Surg Br 1978;60(4):464; with permission.)

second smaller study nor by supplementation after disease onset.[32]

Maternal smoking is a known cause of impaired growth in the fetus. Several studies have attempted to examine a potential relationship, but the only one to do this adequately was based on the Swedish inpatient register. A large case-control study of 852 cases and 4432 controls using linkage to the mother's maternal records concluded that there was a significantly increased risk of Perthes disease with maternal or paternal smoking, with a dose-related effect on risk (adjusted OR 1.4 for <10 cigarettes/day, and OR 2.0 for >10 cigarettes/day)[28] The investigators considered socioeconomic status as a confounder, although it is unclear how this was measured.

Neither of these hypotheses have been satisfactorily resolved one way or the other. The difficulty is that good data and biologic samples are needed from the mother when she is pregnant (for cotinine or trace metal measurements), but the disease is insufficiently common to allow this to be done within existing birth cohorts.

Two other hypotheses relate to postulated later-stage events in the disease pathogenesis. One is hyperactive behavior as a cause of increased trauma to the growing hip, and the second is a coagulation abnormality leading to the vascular occlusion.

Several investigators have commented on behavior abnormalities in their patients with Perthes disease. One study has documented this using standardized validated questionnaires.[33] In a series of 24 children with the disease, 8 had a behavioural profile within the spectrum of the attention deficit hyperactivity disorder (ADHD). However, there were no controls, and this rate was merely compared to the expected population ADHD prevalence of 3% to 5%.

Thrombophilic tendencies have been the subject of a series of studies over the last 15 years, and these have been systematically reviewed. A total of 475 Perthes cases were included in the review by Kenet and colleagues,[34] who concluded that there were no significant differences in antithrombin activity, protein S or C activity, or antiphospholipid antibodies. The review was equivocal over a possible relationship between Perthes disease and the Factor V Leiden mutation, requiring more cases to define the true relationship. The one study since this review included 169 cases of Perthes disease and 512 controls.[35] This study demonstrated several associations including a propensity toward Factor V Leiden mutations (OR 3.3; 95% CI 1.6–6.7) and a raised Factor VIII level (OR 7.5; 95% CI 2.2–25.2). However, this study was so flawed in design

and analysis that it adds nothing to the earlier review.

In terms of these hypotheses, therefore, behavior has not yet been adequately tested and the studies of coagulopathy appear to exclude any major association.

SUMMARY

Perthes disease, despite a century of research, remains of unknown etiology. However, any hypothesis must fit into the clear epidemiologic framework that we have. The disease is associated with deprived populations, and is much more common in white children than in Asians or Africans. It is associated with a global growth disorder characterized by delayed and disproportionate growth. The causal insult appears to occur very early in a child's life, with early changes in skeletal development probably evident at birth. The association with congenital malformations is consistent with this timing. Regarding the incidence of Perthes disease, the strong gradient in social class and the variation in the factors geography and time confirm that the major cause is environmental and not genetic.

Future research is therefore needed to expand our knowledge of descriptive epidemiology; further work on changes in incidence over time would be particularly valuable. Studies are needed to examine the specific hypotheses related to parental smoking, nutritional deficiency in pregnancy, and behavior. However, most urgent are some new hypotheses and adequately designed studies to address them.

REFERENCES

1. Joseph B, Chacko V, Rao BS, et al. The epidemiology of Perthes' disease in south India. Int J Epidemiol 1988;17(3):603–7.
2. Molloy MK, MacMahon B. Incidence of Legg-Perthes disease (osteochondritis deformans). N Engl J Med 1966;275(18):988–90.
3. Gray IM, Lowry RB, Renwick DH. Incidence and genetics of Legg-Perthes disease (osteochondritis deformans) in British Columbia: evidence of polygenic determination. J Med Genet 1972;9(2):197–202.
4. Barker DJ, Dixon E, Taylor JF. Perthes' disease of the hip in three regions of England. J Bone Joint Surg Br 1978;60(4):478–80.
5. Purry NA. The incidence of Perthes' disease in three population groups in the Eastern Cape region of South Africa. J Bone Joint Surg Br 1982;64(3):286–8.
6. Hall AJ, Barker DJ, Dangerfield PH, et al. Perthes' disease of the hip in Liverpool. Br Med J (Clin Res Ed) 1983;287(6407):1757–9.

7. Hall AJ, Barker DJ. Perthes' disease in Yorkshire. J Bone Joint Surg Br 1989;71(2):229–33.

8. Moberg A, Rehnberg L. Incidence of Perthes' disease in Uppsala, Sweden. Acta Orthop Scand 1992;63(2):157–8.

9. Kealey WD, Moore AJ, Cook S, et al. Deprivation, urbanisation and Perthes' disease in Northern Ireland. J Bone Joint Surg Br 2000;82(2):167–71.

10. Margetts BM, Perry CA, Taylor JF, et al. The incidence and distribution of Legg-Calvé-Perthes' disease in Liverpool, 1982–95. Arch Dis Child 2001;84(4):351–4.

11. Rowe SM, Jung ST, Lee KB, et al. The incidence of Perthes' disease in Korea: a focus on differences among races. J Bone Joint Surg Br 2005;87(12):1666–8.

12. Pillai A, Atiya S, Costigan PS. The incidence of Perthes' disease in Southwest Scotland. J Bone Joint Surg Br 2005;87(11):1531–5.

13. Kim W, Hiroshima K, Imaeda T. Multicenter study for Legg-Calvé-Perthes disease in Japan. J Orthop Sci 2006;11(4):333–41.

14. Wiig O, Terjesen T, Svenningsen S, et al. The epidemiology and aetiology of Perthes' disease in Norway. A nationwide study of 425 patients. J Bone Joint Surg Br 2006;88(9):1217–23.

15. Katz JF. Legg-Calve-Perthes disease: a statistical evaluation of 358 cases. Mt Sinai J Med 1973;40(1):20–47.

16. Hall AJ, Barker DJ, Lawton D. The social origins of Perthes' disease of the hip. Paediatr Perinat Epidemiol 1990;4(1):64–70.

17. Sharma S, Sibinski M, Sherlock DA. A profile of Perthes' disease in Greater Glasgow: is there an association with deprivation? J Bone Joint Surg Br 2005;87(11):1536–40.

18. Peic S. Contribution to Perthes' disease. Z Orthop Ihre Grenzgeb 1962;96:276–82.

19. Fisher RL. An epidemiological study of Legg-Perthes disease. J Bone Joint Surg Am 1972;54(4):769–78.

20. Wansbrough R, Carrie A, Walker N, et al. Coxa plana, its genetic aspects and results of treatment with the Long Taylor Walking Caliper: a long-term follow-up study. J Bone Joint Surg Am 1959;41(1):135.

21. Harper PS, Brotherton BJ, Cochlin D. Genetic risks in Perthes' disease. Clin Genet 1976;10(3):178–82.

22. Lappin K, Kealey D, Cosgrove A, et al. Does low birthweight predispose to Perthes' disease? Perthes' disease in twins. J Pediatr Orthop B 2003;12(5):307–10.

23. Wynne-Davies R, Gormley J. The aetiology of Perthes' disease. Genetic, epidemiological and growth factors in 310 Edinburgh and Glasgow patients. J Bone Joint Surg Br 1978;60(1):6–14.

24. Hall AJ, Barker DJ. The age distribution of Legg-Perthes disease. An analysis using Sartwell's incubation period model. Am J Epidemiol 1984;120(4):531–6.

25. Burwell R, Dangerfield P, Hall D, et al. Perthes' disease. An anthropometric study revealing impaired and disproportionate growth. J Bone Joint Surg Br 1978;60:461–77.

26. Hall AJ, Barker DJ, Dangerfield PH, et al. Small feet and Perthes' disease. A survey in Liverpool. J Bone Joint Surg Br 1988;70(4):611–3.

27. Molloy MK, Macmahon B. Birth weight and Legg-Perthes disease. J Bone Joint Surg Am 1967;49(3):498–506.

28. Bahmanyar S, Montgomery SM, Weiss RJ, et al. Maternal smoking during pregnancy, other prenatal and perinatal factors, and the risk of Legg-Calvé-Perthes disease. Pediatrics 2008;122(2):e459–64.

29. Catterall A, Lloyd-Roberts G, Wynne-Davies R. Association of Perthes' disease with congenital anomalies of genitourinary tract and inguinal region. Lancet 1971;297(7707):996–7.

30. Hall DJ, Harrison MH, Burwell RG. Congenital abnormalities and Perthes' disease. Clinical evidence that children with Perthes' disease may have a major congenital defect. J Bone Joint Surg Br 1979;61(1):18–25.

31. Hall AJ, Margetts BM, Barker DJP, et al. Low blood manganese levels in Liverpool children with Perthes' disease. Paediatr Perinat Epidemiol 1989;3(2):131–5.

32. Perry CA, Taylor JF, Nunn A, et al. Perthes disease and blood manganese levels. Arch Dis Child 2000;82(5):428.

33. Loder RT, Schwartz EM, Hensinger RN. Behavioral characteristics of children with Legg-Calvé-Perthes disease. J Pediatr Orthop 1993;13(5):598–601.

34. Kenet G, Ezra E, Wientroub S, et al. Perthes' disease and the search for genetic associations: collagen mutations, Gaucher's disease and thrombophilia. J Bone Joint Surg B 2008;90:1507–11.

35. Vosmaer A, Pereira RR, Koenderman JS, et al. Coagulation abnormalities in Legg-Calvé-Perthes disease. J Bone Joint Surg Am 2010;92(1):121–8.

Pathophysiology, Classifications, and Natural History of Perthes Disease

Harry K.W. Kim, MD, MSc, FRCSC[a,b,*], John A. Herring, MD[b,c]

KEYWORDS

- Legg-Calvé-Perthes disease • Avascular necrosis
- Ischemic necrosis • Pathophysiology • Classifications
- Natural History • Pediatric • Femoral Head

PATHOPHYSIOLOGY

It is generally accepted that a disruption of blood supply to the femoral head is a key pathogenic event in Legg-Calvé-Perthes disease (LCPD). Necropsy and biopsy studies of patients with LCPD show evidence of tissue necrosis consistent with ischemic injury.[1,2] Various imaging studies also show evidence of disruption of blood flow to the affected femoral head.[3–7] Furthermore, the disruption of the blood supply to the femoral head in large animal models (porcine and canine models) produced histopathological and radiographic changes resembling LCPD.[8,9]

The histopathological features of LCPD have been reported in several studies; however, these studies are limited by a small sample size.[1,2,10–16] This limitation underscores one of the major obstacles in trying to understand the pathophysiology of a condition that seems to have so many variables. From the studies that are available, it can be summarized that the pathologic processes in LCPD affect the articular cartilage and the bony epiphysis, and in some patients the metaphysis and the physis.

Pathologic changes in the articular cartilage are mainly observed in the deep layer of the cartilage, which functions as a growth cartilage responsible for the circumferential growth of the bony epiphysis. The damage produces a cessation of endochondral ossification at the cartilage-subchondral bone junction. Other changes, including separation of cartilage from underlying subchondral bone, vascular invasion of the cartilage, and new accessory ossification, have been observed in various stages of LCPD.[1,2] In the bony epiphysis, the necrosis of the marrow space and the trabecular bone, compression fracture of trabeculae, osteoclastic resorption, fibrovascular granulation tissue invasion of the necrotic head, and thickened trabeculae have been reported in various stages of LCPD. The physeal changes are most often seen in the anterior aspect of the femoral head, with areas of growth plate cartilage extending below the endochondral ossification line. Premature growth arrest is seen in fewer than 30% of patients with LCPD, suggesting that in a majority of the patients the growth plate continues to function.[17,18] Metaphyseal changes are commonly seen during the early stages of LCPD, usually found below the growth plate.[19,20] The mechanisms responsible for the appearance of these lesions are unclear. Various tissue types have been reported, including columns of normal or degenerated cartilage extending down to the

No funding was received for this work.
The authors have nothing to disclose.

[a] Center for Excellence in Hip Disorders, Research Department, Texas Scottish Rite Hospital for Children, 2222 Welborn Street, Dallas, TX 75219, USA
[b] Department of Orthopaedic Surgery, UT Southwestern Medical Center, 1801 Inwood Road, Dallas, TX 75390, USA
[c] Texas Scottish Rite Hospital for Children, 2222 Welborn Street, Dallas, TX 75219, USA
* Corresponding author. Texas Scottish Rite Hospital for Children, 2222 Welborn Street, Dallas, TX 75219.
E-mail address: harry.kim@tsrh.org

Orthop Clin N Am 42 (2011) 285–295
doi:10.1016/j.ocl.2011.04.007

metaphysis, fibrocartilage, fat necrosis, vascular proliferation, and focal fibrosis.[1,21] Some have found an association between the presence of radiolucent metaphyseal changes and poor prognosis[19,22,23] whereas others have not.[24]

Experimental Studies

Further insight into the pathophysiology of ischemic necrosis in the immature femoral head and also the temporal evolution of histopathological changes over time has been gained using an experimental model of ischemic necrosis (piglet model) (**Fig. 1**).[8,21,25–28] After the induction of ischemic necrosis in immature pigs by ligating the femoral neck blood vessels, the earliest histologic changes are seen in the marrow space with diffuse cell death, disorganization of the marrow stroma, and the loss of osteoblasts lining the trabecular bone. The mechanisms of cell death appear to involve apoptosis and necrosis.[29] Empty lacunae, a classic feature of osteonecrosis, are seen in the necrotic bone within a few weeks.

Along with the necrosis of the bony epiphysis, cell death is observed in the deep layer the articular cartilage, which is similar to the findings in cartilage from histopathological studies of LCPD.[26,30,31] The reason for the cell death is that the articular cartilage of the immature femoral head is thicker than that of the adult articular cartilage, and its deep layer is dependent on the subchondral vascularity for nutritional support.[26,32–34] Because of this dependence, a loss of blood supply to the immature femoral head not only produces a necrotic damage to the bony epiphysis but also damage to the deep layer of the articular cartilage surrounding the secondary center of ossification.[14,26] The consequence is a growth arrest of the secondary center, which is an early radiographic feature of the piglet model and LCPD. One significant implication of this damage is a potential for growth disturbance of the secondary center.[26] Unless the restoration of growth of the secondary center is symmetric, restoring a spherical growth, a further deformity of the femoral head can ensue with asymmetric restoration of the growth. This process occurs in addition to the potential growth disturbance of the metaphyseal physis, which is responsible for the length and the alignment of the femoral neck (coxa breva, coxa vara, or coxa valga).[35,36] In the piglet model, disruption of blood flow to the epiphysis produced limited damage to the metaphyseal physis.[21,25] In most of the animals the growth plate continued to function, albeit at a slower rate than the growth plate on the normal side, indicating that femoral head ischemia does not necessarily produce a growth arrest of the metaphyseal physis.

Revascularization and healing of the necrotic femoral head in immature pigs come in the form of fibrovascular tissue invasion of the necrotic marrow space and resorption of the necrotic bone.[8] The new vessels arise from the existing vessels on the femoral neck, which invade through the periphery of the cartilage to reach the necrotic secondary center.[30] In general, the invading vessels do not cross the metaphyseal physis. The fibrovascular tissue consists of inflammatory, mesenchymal (fibroblast-like in appearance), osteoclasts, and endothelial cells. In the revascularized regions of the bone, increased osteoclast-mediated resorption is observed with a net loss of bone, due to the imbalance of bone resorption and formation.[8] The necrotic bone is replaced by a fibrovascular tissue, and bone formation is noticeably absent in these areas. Radiographic and histologic findings in the piglet model at this stage of healing resemble the fragmentation stage in LCPD, at which resorptive changes in the necrotic bone predominate while reossification of the resorbed areas is delayed for many months.

Pathogenesis of Femoral Head Deformity

The pathogenesis of the femoral head deformity in the immature femoral head is complex. From a mechanical perspective, the infarcted femoral head begins to deform when the forces applied to the femoral head due to loading are greater than its ability to resist deformation (**Fig. 2**). While it is clear that osteonecrosis induces mechanical weakening of the femoral head, the mechanisms involved with the process are only beginning to be elucidated. Experimental studies in a large animal model of ischemic necrosis found a significant decrease in the mechanical properties of the infarcted femoral head and its components (articular cartilage and bone) from an early stage of the model.[27,28] These studies, along with recent study on the alteration of calcium content of the necrotic bone,[37] suggest that the mechanical properties of the infarcted femoral head are compromised by various mechanisms at different stages of the disease. In the early stage (avascular stage), before the initiation of revascularization, increased calcium content of the necrotic bone is thought to increase the brittleness of the necrotic bone and make it more prone to microdamage.[37] In the absence of bone cells, such as osteoblasts, osteocytes, and osteoclasts, due to necrosis, the microfractures remain undetected and unrepaired, and accumulate. It is proposed that the accumulation of microdamage incurred with normal activities compromise the mechanical properties of the femoral head in the early stages of LCPD,

Proposed Pathogenesis of Femoral Head Deformity Following Ischemic Necrosis

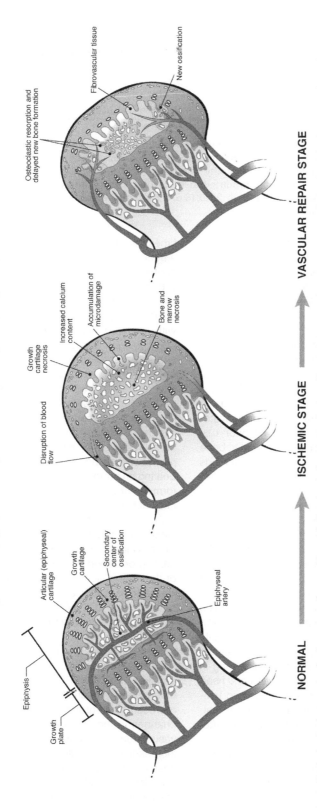

Fig. 1. Pathologic changes in the immature femoral head following ischemic necrosis. Ischemic injury produces extensive cell death in the bony epiphysis (osteonecrosis) and the deep layer of the articular cartilage (chondronecrosis). The deep layer of the cartilage represents the growth cartilage responsible for the circumferential growth of the secondary center of ossification. The ischemic damage to the deep layer of the cartilage produces a growth arrest of the secondary center. Ischemic necrosis is also associated with an increased calcium content of the necrotic bone, which is thought to make the bone more brittle and more prone to microdamage accumulation with hip joint loading. Revascularization of the infarcted femoral head is associated with a predominance of osteoclast-mediated resorption and a delayed bone formation, which further contribute to the development of the femoral head deformity. (*Courtesy of* Texas Scottish Rite Hospital for Children; with permission.)

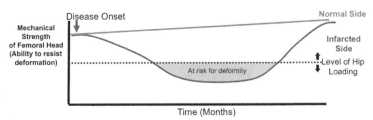

Proposed Pathogenesis of Femoral Head Deformity

Fig. 2. A line graph representing proposed mechanical changes in the necrotic femoral head. The extent of head involvement, the degree of imbalance between bone resorption and formation, the duration of healing, and the level of hip loading will likely affect the deformity. The potential to remodel the deformed head, as seen in young patients, will offset the deformity produced at the acute phase of the disease. (*From* Kim HK. Legg-Calvé-Perthes Disease. J Am Acad Orthop Surg 2010;18:676–86; with permission. Copyright © 2010 American Academy of Orthopaedic Surgeons.)

and lead to the development of a subchondral fracture and compression fracture of the superior region of the bony epiphysis.

Vascular invasion and subsequent resorption of the necrotic bone seen at the vascular stage of healing further compromise the mechanical properties of the infarcted head.[28] Experimental studies show that the imbalance of bone resorption and formation with a predominance of resorption contributes significantly to the pathogenesis of the femoral head deformity.[8] Experimental studies also show that inhibition of bone resorption using bisphosphonates or a RANKL (receptor activator of nuclear factor kappa-B ligand) inhibitor can improve the preservation of the trabecular bone and the femoral head shape.[38–42] These findings support the hypothesis that osteoclast-mediated bone resorption is a significant contributor to the pathogenesis of femoral head deformity. Although there are a few studies on the use of bisphosphonate to treat femoral head osteonecrosis in children,[43–45] the efficacy of this treatment for LCPD has not been investigated.

Because the hip joint is a major load-bearing joint and children with LCPD tend to be active, it is important to consider the potential role of hip joint loading on the development of the femoral head deformity. This area of LCPD research is one that has a paucity of data. Basic data such as the hip contact pressures associated with various activities of daily living in children are not available. In adults, a femoral head prosthesis equipped with a strain gauge and telemetric transmission capability has allowed a real-time collection of femoral head loading data after total hip replacement while the patients were performing various activities and positioning of the affected leg.[46] The measurements indicated that substantial forces act on the femoral head with weight-bearing activities. Walking was associated with the hip contact pressure reaching about 2.5

times the body weight with each step. Running on a treadmill at a rate of 8 km per hour increased the contact pressure to about 4.5 times the body weight with each stride. Greater pressures are generated with faster speeds of walking or running. Some supine and prone activities were also associated with elevated hip contact pressures above the body weight. Direct measurements of the hip contact pressures are not available in children; however, children in general are more active and take more steps, taking on average 7500 steps per day.[47] In a disease where femoral head deformity is produced because of mechanical weakening, avoidance of activities that generate high hip contact pressures would seem reasonable. While some retrospective studies support the role of non–weight bearing on protecting the femoral head from the deforming forces,[48] the compliance and the true efficacy of this type of treatment remain unclear.

In contrast to the factors such as femoral head weakening and hip joint loading that may promote the development of femoral head deformity, the healing or remodeling potential related to the age of the patient seems to offset the deformity. Clinical studies show a better outcome in younger patients with LCPD (onset of disease before age 6 years) compared with older patients (onset of disease after age 8 years).[49] The mechanisms responsible for the difference in healing are unclear. One important age-related factor to consider is that LCPD affects a wide age range of children (preschool to teenage years), which represents a growth period when significant changes in the femoral head anatomy, size, and vasculature are occurring.[50–53] The bony epiphysis increases in size while the articular cartilage thickness and the growth potential of the bony epiphysis decrease with age. Other changes, such as the regression of cartilage canals (blood vessels within cartilage) and the changes in the vascular anatomy of the proximal femur, are also occurring. As these changes are taking place, the onset of the disease at different ages implies that the disease is affecting a femoral head that may have significantly different growth and remodeling potentials that could affect the outcome of the femoral head. Preliminary experimental studies suggest that the potential for femoral head healing may be greater in the younger animals than in older, immature animals, and that one of the mechanisms may be related to greater hypoxic and angiogenic repair responses generated in the femoral head cartilage of the younger animals.[54]

CLASSIFICATIONS

The classifications for LCPD can be divided into the one that defines the stage of the disease and the ones used to prognosticate outcome. Waldenström's radiographic classification defines 4 radiographic stages of LCPD during the active phase of the disease, termed the initial stage, fragmentation stage, reossification stage, and residual stage, according to the characteristic radiographic features of each stage (**Table 1**). The duration of each stage is variable from one patient to another. What determines the duration of each stage and the total duration of the active phase is unknown. In general, older patients appear to have a longer duration than younger patients. According to one study, the fragmentation staging lasts about 1 year while the reossification stage lasts from 3 to 5 years.[55]

Three radiographic classification systems, namely the Catterall, Salter-Thompson, and lateral pillar, have been developed as prognosticators of outcome that are to be applied at the stage of fragmentation. The Salter-Thompson classification is a two-category system (group A or group B) based on the extent of subchondral fracture (crescent sign).[56] In group A, less than half of the femoral head is involved whereas in group B, more than half of the femoral head is involved. Because the crescent sign can be observed at the initial or early fragmentation stage, it has the advantage of being applicable at an earlier time point than the other 2 systems, which are applicable at the stage of maximal fragmentation. Its application, however, is restricted by the absence of the crescent sign in many patients at the time of presentation and subsequent follow-up. The presence of the sign may also be transient and have a narrow window for detection.

The Catterall classification system is a 4-category system (groups I–IV), and the first to emphasize the relationship between the extent of head involvement and the outcome.[57] The Catterall groups I, II, III, and IV represent 25%, 50%, 75%, and total head involvement, respectively. The system was developed to be applied during the fragmentation stage when the necrotic sequestrum becomes well demarcated from the viable segment of the femoral head. Along with his classification system, Catterall also described head-at-risk signs associated with a poor outcome discussed earlier.[22] The major

Table 1
Waldenstrom's radiographic stages of LCPD

Stages of LCPD	Radiographic Features
Initial stage (stage of increased radiodensity)	Smaller ossific nucleus Increased radiodensity of the ossific nucleus Widening of medial joint space Subchondral fracture in some Metaphyseal cyst in some Mild flattening of the ossific nucleus
Fragmentation stage (resorptive stage)	Appearance of radiolucencies in the ossific nucleus Fragmented appearance of the ossific nucleus Further flattening of the ossific nucleus Further lateralization of the head Demarcation of central radiodense fragment ("sequestrum") from the medial and lateral pillars of the head in some versus whole head flattening in others Some show minimal fragmentation and flattening
Reossification stage (healing stage)	Appearance of new bone in the medial and lateral aspects of the femoral head Central and anterior aspects of the head are last to reossify Disappearance of radiodense fragment Some show improvement of head shape while few show worsening of head shape
Residual stage (healed stage)	Normal radiodensity of the femoral head Shape of the femoral head may change until skeletal maturity

criticism for the Catterall classification system has been its poor interobserver reliability.[58,59] Recently, a modified Catterall classification system with two categories (the groups I and II combined and the groups III and IV combined) has been shown to have a better interobserver reliability.[59] Because the groups I and II are often associated with good outcome and the groups III and IV with poor outcome, the simplification seems reasonable.

The lateral pillar classification was originally designed as a 3-category system (groups A, B, or C) with a recent addition of group B/C border, making this a 4-category system (**Fig. 3**).[60,61] The system is based on the height of the lateral pillar, defined as the lateral 15% to 30% of the epiphysis. Group A represents no loss of the lateral pillar height, whereas group B represents less than 50% loss and group C more than 50% loss of the lateral pillar height. Because the lateral aspect of the femoral head is a site of new ossification, it does pose an uncertainty of what is actually being assessed anatomically in some cases: the collapsed lateral pillar or the new ossification in the lateral aspect of the femoral head. Regardless of this uncertainty, the classification system does reflect the extent of the femoral head deformity, and the 3-category lateral pillar classification has been shown to have better interobserver reliability than the Salter-Thompson and Catterall classification systems.[58,59] It has also been reported to be a better predictor of a Stulberg radiographic outcome than the Catterall classification.[58]

Because the Catterall and lateral pillar classification systems are applicable at the stage of

maximal fragmentation when the femoral head deformity is at its peak, the timing poses a dilemma for those patients seen at the initial stage or at the early fragmentation stage when the femoral head cannot be correctly classified. Assignment of the lateral pillar classification based on the initial presenting radiographs was found to be unreliable in 92 of 275 hips (33%), as the hips showed worsening of the lateral pillar height over time (**Fig. 4**).[62] One treatment approach for the patients presenting in the early stages of the disease has been to wait and observe until the patient can be classified into one of the guarded prognostic groups, either Catterall groups III or IV or lateral pillar groups B, B/C, or C, before instituting a specific treatment. The idea of "wait-and-classify" is a concern for older patients (>8 years old), who are known to have a limited potential to remodel the deformed femoral head, as a significant deformity can develop during this wait and see period. An argument for the "wait-and-classify" approach is that it may prevent having to operate on patients who would not have needed surgery (Catterall group I or II or lateral pillar group A) or who would not have benefited from it (lateral pillar C). An argument against this approach is that the treatment should be instituted early in the older patients rather than waiting for the head to deform, because they do not have as much remodeling potential as the younger patients.[63,64] This controversy highlights the limitations of these radiographic classification systems, which cannot be applied in the early stages of LCPD prior to the development of the femoral head deformity. There

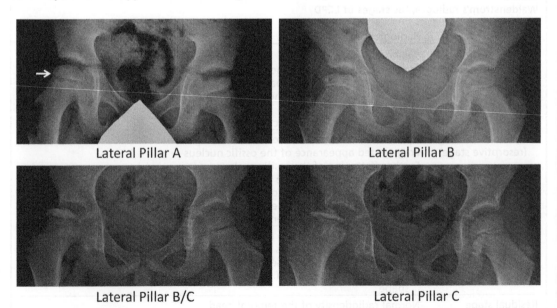

Lateral Pillar A

Lateral Pillar B

Lateral Pillar B/C

Lateral Pillar C

Fig. 3. Examples of lateral pillar classification. The upper left radiograph shows bilateral femoral head involvement with the right femoral head (*white arrow*) classified as a lateral pillar group A.

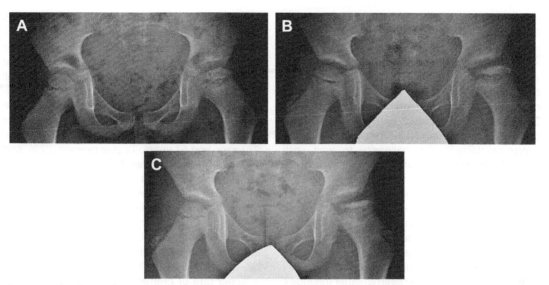

Fig. 4. Serial radiographs of a 7-year-old patient obtained at the time of presentation (*A*), at 3 months' follow-up (*B*), and at 6 months' follow-up (*C*). Application of the lateral pillar classification too early (at the initial or early fragmentation stage) would have led to an incorrect assignment of the lateral pillar group for this patient as B or B/C border at the 3-month follow-up (*B*). A subsequent follow-up at maximal fragmentation stage (*C*) showed that the affected hip was in the lateral pillar group C.

is clearly a need to develop an earlier prognostic indicator based on a more sensitive imaging modality, such as a magnetic resonance image, which can be applied before the deformity develops to guide treatment from the initial stage of the disease. An additional limitation of the current classification systems is that they may not be relevant for older patients (>12 years), who tend to have poor prognosis regardless of the extent of head or lateral pillar involvement.[65]

The Stulberg classification of radiographic outcome is a 5-class system designed to be applied at skeletal maturity to prognosticate the long-term outcome of the affected hip joint. The classification categorizes the severity of the femoral head deformity and the loss of hip joint congruence at maturity. Higher classes (class III, IV, and V hips) had high risk of developing radiographic signs of premature osteoarthritis at 40 years' follow-up (**Table 2**). The risk of developing premature osteoarthritis was substantially less in the spherical femoral heads (class I or II hips). One of the weaknesses of the classification is low to moderate intraobserver and interobserver reliability.[66] The reliability issue is partly related to the qualitative description of the categories, which

Table 2
Stulberg radiographic classification and osteoarthritis at 40 years' follow-up

Stulberg Class	Descriptive Features	Radiographic Signs of Osteoarthritis at the Mean Follow-Up of 40 Years	Radiographic Evidence of Joint Space Narrowing at the Mean Follow-Up of 40 Years
I	Normal hip joint	0	0
II	Spherical head with enlargement, short neck, or steep acetabulum	16%	0
III	Nonspherical head (ovoid, mushroom, or umbrella shaped)	58%	47%
IV	Flat head	75%	53%
V	Flat head with incongruent hip joint	78%	61%

From Stulberg SD, Cooperman DR, Wallensten R. The natural history of Legg-Calvé-Perthes disease. J Bone Joint Surg Am 1981;63:1095; with permission.

is prone to subjective interpretation. A clear distinction between class III and class IV hips is particularly challenging in some cases. Improvements in intraobserver and interobserver reliability (average weighted kappa value of 0.82 and 0.88, respectively) have been reported by assigning numerical criteria for defining the femoral head deformity.[60] Decreasing the number of categories from a 5-class to 3-class system also improved the interobserver reliability.[67] The necessity to wait until skeletal maturity to determine the Stulberg class is another limitation of this outcome system. Recently, the deformity index has been reported as a continuous outcome measure of femoral head deformity that can predict the Stulberg outcome at 2 years into the disease course.[68] The index measures the changes in the femoral epiphyseal height and width in comparison with the unaffected side. It remains to be seen whether this index proves to be a reliable indicator of outcome by other investigators and in prospective studies.

NATURAL HISTORY

Long-term studies on the natural history of the disease are few in number and have limitations due to a small sample size, loss of follow-up, and inclusion of patients treated with various nonoperative treatments that may have influenced their outcome. In general, long-term studies with an average follow-up of less than 40 years show that the majority of the patients are active and asymptomatic even with a deformed femoral head. A study of a cohort from Iowa by Gower and Johnston[69] with an average follow-up of 36 years (range 30–48 years) showed that 6 out of the 36 had surgical procedure(s) as an adult (diagnostic biopsy, subtrochanteric osteotomy, bone grafting of the femoral head, or cup arthroplasty). In the remaining 30 patients, the typical patient had a mild limp, minimum shortening, absent or mild hip pain, and minimum or no functional impairment with respect to job and activities of daily living. The average Iowa hip rating score was 91 points for the cohort. Those with round femoral heads had better hip ratings than those with flattened heads (average 97 points compared with 89 points). Despite good hip ratings, 25% of the patients were found to have radiographic evidence of moderate to severe degenerative arthritis. In longer follow-up studies, noticeable deterioration of hip function has been reported. A study by McAndrew and Weinstein[70] of the cohort from Iowa with an average follow-up of 47 years (range 39–64 years) found that only 40% of the patients maintained a good level of function (a rating >80 points). While 40% already had an arthroplasty at the time of follow-up, an additional

10% had disabling pain, and the remaining 10% had an Iowa hip rating of less than 80 points. Statistically significant correlations were observed between the long-term outcome and age at onset of the disease, femoral head size ratio, ant Catterall head-at-risk signs; however, the Catterall classification alone did not correlate well with the outcome.[70] Mose[71] studied 3 groups of patients with Perthes with an average follow-up of 17 years, 27 years, and 57 years. Twelve percent, 22%, and 100% of the femoral heads with irregular shapes at healing had severe radiographic evidence of osteoarthritis at the average of 17, 27, and 57 years' follow-up. The relationship between the degree of femoral head deformity at skeletal maturity and the long-term risk for developing osteoarthritis is further supported by the findings from the study by Stulberg and colleagues,[72] which showed a higher rate of premature osteoarthritis in those patients with an aspherical femoral head and a greater deformity (Stulberg class III, IV, and V hips).

Age at onset of the disease is an important variable that has consistently been shown to affect the outcome. A majority of the patients with the onset of the disease before age 6 years had a spherical femoral head at skeletal maturity despite receiving nonspecific, symptomatic treatments.[49] Patients older than 8 years at the onset of the disease have a poorer prognosis.[70,73]

SUMMARY

LCPD remains a controversial condition in pediatric orthopedics. Several key questions relating to its pathophysiology, classifications, and natural history remain partially answered. Experimental studies reveal that mechanical and biological factors contribute to the pathophysiology of the femoral head deformity following ischemic necrosis. Further research is needed to define the mechanisms responsible for the pathologic healing process and how to control the process effectively. This research will lead to development of new treatments based on the pathophysiology of the disease. Going forward, there is also a need to develop early prognostic indicators that can be applied before the development of the femoral head deformity. These improvements will allow orthopedists to better define who to treat, when to treat, and with what to treat.

REFERENCES

1. Catterall A, Pringle J, Byers PD, et al. A review of the morphology of Perthes' disease. J Bone Joint Surg Br 1982;64:269.

2. Jonsater S. Coxa plana; a histo-pathologic and arthrographic study. Acta Orthop Scand Suppl 1953;12:5.

3. Atsumi T, Yamano K, Muraki M, et al. The blood supply of the lateral epiphyseal arteries in Perthes' disease. J Bone Joint Surg Br 2000;82:392.

4. Conway JJ. A scintigraphic classification of Legg-Calvé-Perthes disease. Semin Nucl Med 1993;23:274.

5. de Camargo FP, de Godoy RM Jr, Tovo R. Angiography in Perthes' disease. Clin Orthop Relat Res 1984;(191):216.

6. Lamer S, Dorgeret S, Khairouni A, et al. Femoral head vascularisation in Legg-Calvé-Perthes disease: comparison of dynamic gadolinium-enhanced subtraction MRI with bone scintigraphy. Pediatr Radiol 2002;32:580.

7. Theron J. Angiography in Legg-Calvé-Perthes disease. Radiology 1980;135:81.

8. Kim HK, Su PH. Development of flattening and apparent fragmentation following ischemic necrosis of the capital femoral epiphysis in a piglet model. J Bone Joint Surg Am 2002;84:1329.

9. Sanchis M, Zahir A, Freeman MA. The experimental simulation of Perthes disease by consecutive interruptions of the blood supply to the capital femoral epiphysis in the puppy. J Bone Joint Surg Am 1973;55:335.

10. Catterall A, Pringle J, Byers PD, et al. Perthes' disease: is the epiphyseal infarction complete? J Bone Joint Surg Br 1982;64:276.

11. Dolman CL, Bell HM. The pathology of Legg-Calvé-Perthes disease. A case report. J Bone Joint Surg Am 1973;55:184.

12. Inoue A, Freeman MA, Vernon-Roberts B, et al. The pathogenesis of Perthes' disease. J Bone Joint Surg Br 1976;58:453.

13. McKibbin B, Ralis Z. Pathological changes in a case of Perthes' disease. J Bone Joint Surg Br 1974; 56B:438.

14. Milgram JW. Idiopathic osteonecrosis of the juvenile femoral head (Legg-Calvé-Perthes disease). In: Radiologic and histologic pathology of nontumorous diseases of bones and joints, vol. 2. Northbrook (IL): Northbrook Publishing Company; 1990. p. 1093.

15. Ponseti IV. Legg-Perthes disease; observations on pathological changes in two cases. J Bone Joint Surg Am 1956;38:739.

16. Ponseti IV, Maynard JA, Weinstein SL, et al. Legg-Calvé-Perthes disease. Histochemical and ultrastructural observations of the epiphyseal cartilage and physis. J Bone Joint Surg Am 1983;65:797.

17. Bowen JR, Schreiber FC, Foster BK, et al. Premature femoral neck physeal closure in Perthes' disease. Clin Orthop Relat Res 1982;(171):24.

18. Sponseller PD, Desai SS, Millis MB. Abnormalities of proximal femoral growth after severe Perthes' disease. J Bone Joint Surg Br 1989;71:610.

19. Katz JF, Siffert RS. Capital necrosis, metaphyseal cyst and subluxation in coxa plana. Clin Orthop Relat Res 1975;(106):75.

20. Smith SR, Ions GK, Gregg PJ. The radiological features of the metaphysis in Perthes disease. J Pediatr Orthop 1982;2:401.

21. Kim HK, Skelton DN, Quigley EJ. Pathogenesis of metaphyseal radiolucent changes following ischemic necrosis of the capital femoral epiphysis in immature pigs. A preliminary report. J Bone Joint Surg Am 2004;86:129.

22. Catterall A. Legg-Calvé-Perthes syndrome. Clin Orthop Relat Res 1981;(158):41.

23. Yrjonen T, Poussa M, Hoikka V, et al. Poor prognosis in atypical Perthes' disease. Radiographic analysis of 19 hips after 35 years. Acta Orthop Scand 1992;63:399.

24. Mukherjee A, Fabry G. Evaluation of the prognostic indices in Legg-Calvé-Perthes disease: statistical analysis of 116 hips. J Pediatr Orthop 1990;10:153.

25. Kim HK, Stephenson N, Garces A, et al. Effects of disruption of epiphyseal vasculature on the proximal femoral growth plate. J Bone Joint Surg Am 2009; 91:1149.

26. Kim HK, Su PH, Qiu YS. Histopathologic changes in growth-plate cartilage following ischemic necrosis of the capital femoral epiphysis. An experimental investigation in immature pigs. J Bone Joint Surg Am 2001;83:688.

27. Koob TJ, Pringle D, Gedbaw E, et al. Biomechanical properties of bone and cartilage in growing femoral head following ischemic osteonecrosis. J Orthop Res 2007;25:750.

28. Pringle D, Koob TJ, Kim HK. Indentation properties of growing femoral head following ischemic necrosis. J Orthop Res 2004;22:122.

29. Kothapalli R, Aya-ay JP, Bian H, et al. Ischaemic injury to femoral head induces apoptotic and oncotic cell death. Pathology 2007;39:241.

30. Kim HK, Bian H, Aya-ay J, et al. Hypoxia and HIF-1alpha expression in the epiphyseal cartilage following ischemic injury to the immature femoral head. Bone 2009;45:280.

31. Kim HK, Bian H, Randall T, et al. Increased VEGF expression in the epiphyseal cartilage after ischemic necrosis of the capital femoral epiphysis. J Bone Miner Res 2004;19:2041.

32. Carlson CS, Meulen DJ, Richardson DC. Ischemic necrosis of cartilage in spontaneous and experimental lesions of osteochondrosis. J Orthop Res 1991;9:317.

33. McKibbin B, Holdsworth FW. The nutrition of immature joint cartilage in the lamb. J Bone Joint Surg Br 1966;48:793.

34. Ytrehus B, Andreas Haga H, Mellum CN, et al. Experimental ischemia of porcine growth cartilage produces lesions of osteochondrosis. J Orthop Res 2004;22:1201.

35. Kalamchi A, MacEwen GD. Avascular necrosis following treatment of congenital dislocation of the hip. J Bone Joint Surg Am 1980;62:876.

36. Salter RB, Kostuik J, Dallas S. Avascular necrosis of the femoral head as a complication of treatment for congenital dislocation of the hip in young children: a clinical and experimental investigation. Can J Surg 1969;12:44.

37. Hofstaetter JG, Roschger P, Klaushofer K, et al. Increased matrix mineralization in the immature femoral head following ischemic osteonecrosis. Bone 2010;46:379.

38. Aya-ay J, Athavale S, Morgan-Bagley S, et al. Retention, distribution, and effects of intraosseously administered ibandronate in the infarcted femoral head. J Bone Miner Res 2007;22:93.

39. Kim HK, Morgan-Bagley S, Kostenuik P. RANKL inhibition: a novel strategy to decrease femoral head deformity after ischemic osteonecrosis. J Bone Miner Res 1946;21:2006.

40. Kim HK, Randall TS, Bian H, et al. Ibandronate for prevention of femoral head deformity after ischemic necrosis of the capital femoral epiphysis in immature pigs. J Bone Joint Surg Am 2005;87: 550.

41. Little DG, McDonald M, Sharpe IT, et al. Zoledronic acid improves femoral head sphericity in a rat model of Perthes disease. J Orthop Res 2005;23:862.

42. Little DG, Peat RA, McEvoy A, et al. Zoledronic acid treatment results in retention of femoral head structure after traumatic osteonecrosis in young Wistar rats. J Bone Miner Res 2003;18: 2016.

43. Kotecha RS, Powers N, Lee SJ, et al. Use of bisphosphonates for the treatment of osteonecrosis as a complication of therapy for childhood acute lymphoblastic leukaemia (ALL). Pediatr Blood Cancer 2010;54:934.

44. Nguyen T, Zacharin MR. Pamidronate treatment of steroid associated osteonecrosis in young patients treated for acute lymphoblastic leukaemia—two-year outcomes. J Pediatr Endocrinol Metab 2006; 19:161.

45. Ramachandran M, Ward K, Brown RR, et al. Intravenous bisphosphonate therapy for traumatic osteonecrosis of the femoral head in adolescents. J Bone Joint Surg Am 2007;89:1727.

46. Bergmann G, Deuretzbacher G, Heller M, et al. Hip contact forces and gait patterns from routine activities. J Biomech 2001;34:859.

47. Song KM, Bjornson KF, Cappello T, et al. Use of the StepWatch activity monitor for characterization of normal activity levels of children. J Pediatr Orthop 2006;26:245.

48. Kuroda T, Mitani S, Sugimoto Y, et al. Changes in the lateral pillar classification in Perthes' disease. J Pediatr Orthop B 2009;18:116.

49. Rosenfeld SB, Herring JA, Chao JC. Legg-Calvé-Perthes disease: a review of cases with onset before six years of age. J Bone Joint Surg Am 2007;89: 2712.

50. Chung SM. The arterial supply of the developing proximal end of the human femur. J Bone Joint Surg Am 1976;58:961.

51. Meszaros T, Kery L. Quantitative analysis of the growth of the hip joint. A radiological study. Acta Orthop Scand 1980;51:275.

52. Ogden JA. Changing patterns of proximal femoral vascularity. J Bone Joint Surg Am 1974;56:941.

53. Trueta J. The normal vascular anatomy of the human femoral head during growth. J Bone Joint Surg Br 1957;39:358.

54. Kim H, Bian H, Aya-ay J, et al. Age affects hypoxia and hypoxia-inducible factor-1 (HIF-1) level in the epiphyseal cartilage following ischemic injury to the immature femoral head. J Bone Miner Res 2009;24(Suppl 1):SU0015.

55. Herring JA, Williams JJ, Neustadt JN, et al. Evolution of femoral head deformity during the healing phase of Legg-Calvé-Perthes disease. J Pediatr Orthop 1993;13:41.

56. Salter RB, Thompson GH. Legg-Calvé-Perthes disease. The prognostic significance of the subchondral fracture and a two-group classification of the femoral head involvement. J Bone Joint Surg Am 1984;66:479.

57. Catterall A. The natural history of Perthes' disease. J Bone Joint Surg Br 1971;53:37.

58. Ritterbusch JF, Shantharam SS, Gelinas C. Comparison of lateral pillar classification and Catterall classification of Legg-Calvé-Perthes' disease. J Pediatr Orthop 1993;13:200.

59. Wiig O, Terjesen T, Svenningsen S. Inter-observer reliability of radiographic classifications and measurements in the assessment of Perthes' disease. Acta Orthop Scand 2002;73:523.

60. Herring JA, Kim HT, Browne R. Legg-Calvé-Perthes disease. Part I: classification of radiographs with use of the modified lateral pillar and Stulberg classifications. J Bone Joint Surg Am 2004;86:2103.

61. Herring JA, Neustadt JB, Williams JJ, et al. The lateral pillar classification of Legg-Calvé-Perthes disease. J Pediatr Orthop 1992;12:143.

62. Lappin K, Kealey D, Cosgrove A. Herring classification: how useful is the initial radiograph? J Pediatr Orthop 2002;22:479.

63. Little DG. Legg-Calvé-Perthes disease: the effect of treatment on outcome. J Bone Joint Surg Am 2005; 87:1164.

64. Price CT. The lateral pillar classification for Legg-Calvé-Perthes disease. J Pediatr Orthop 2007;27: 592.

65. Joseph B, Mulpuri K, Varghese G. Perthes' disease in the adolescent. J Bone Joint Surg Br 2001;83:715.

66. Neyt JG, Weinstein SL, Spratt KF, et al. Stulberg classification system for evaluation of Legg-Calvé-Perthes disease: intra-rater and inter-rater reliability. J Bone Joint Surg Am 1999;81:1209.

67. Wiig O, Terjesen T, Svenningsen S. Inter-observer reliability of the Stulberg classification in the assessment of Perthes disease. J Child Orthop 2007;1:101.

68. Nelson D, Zenios M, Ward K, et al. The deformity index as a predictor of final radiological outcome in Perthes' disease. J Bone Joint Surg Br 2007;89:1369.

69. Gower WE, Johnston RC. Legg-Perthes disease. Long-term follow-up of thirty-six patients. J Bone Joint Surg Am 1971;53:759.

70. McAndrew MP, Weinstein SL. A long-term follow-up of Legg-Calvé-Perthes disease. J Bone Joint Surg Am 1984;66:860.

71. Mose K. Methods of measuring in Legg-Calvé-Perthes disease with special regard to the prognosis. Clin Orthop Relat Res 1980;(150):103.

72. Stulberg SD, Cooperman DR, Wallensten R. The natural history of Legg-Calvé-Perthes disease. J Bone Joint Surg Am 1981;63:1095.

73. Herring JA, Kim HT, Browne R. Legg-Calvé-Perthes disease. Part II: prospective multicenter study of the effect of treatment on outcome. J Bone Joint Surg Am 2004;86:2121.

Imaging in Legg-Calvé-Perthes Disease

Alain Dimeglio, MD[a], Federico Canavese, MD, PhD[b],*

KEYWORDS

- Legg-Calvé-Perthes disease • Radiography
- Magnetic resonance imaging • Computed tomography
- Scintigraphy • Arthrography

Imaging in Legg-Calvé-Perthes (LCP) disease should help assess the severity and the stage of the disease, detect severe forms early, and provide guidance to therapy. However, due to the complexity of the disease, not all examinations can be performed at the same time and with the same results.[1–5]

This article aims to provide answers to 3 basic questions:

1. What is the optimal imaging technique to evaluate patients with LCP disease?
2. What is the correlation between different imaging techniques?
3. Which technique allows the surgeon to anticipate the changes induced by the disease, to provide early containment and, eventually, better outcome?

IMAGING

Several imaging techniques are available and possible. Each technique has advantages and disadvantages.

Plain Radiographs

It is generally accepted that it is best to initiate imaging of LCP disease with anteroposterior (AP) and frog lateral plain radiographs, and to image both hips to detect any contralateral disease (**Fig. 1**).

Plain radiographs are used to assess the stage, extent, and severity of the femoral head involvement, and also the stage of the clinical course. Three radiographic classifications are currently used with the aim of identifying patients with poorer outcome. However, radiographic classifications have the disadvantage that is difficult to use during the early phases of the disease. Overall, radiologic classifications provide useful retrospective insight into treatment options and may help guide the treatment of some patients. However, there is still a need for a prospective prognostic indicator to assist decision making in the early stages of LCP disease, when outcome can be influenced.[6–10]

To have some positive effects on femoral head reconstruction, surgical treatment should be started during the initial or the early fragmentation phase. Anticipation is the best strategy.[5] Unfortunately, radiographic changes become evident about 3 to 4 months after their actual onset, and standard radiographic findings may be entirely normal in early symptomatic disease; in particular, LCP disease can be radiographically silent during the first 3 to 6 months.[11–17]

Catterall classification (1971)

Catterall established a radiologic classification that utilizes AP and lateral radiographs and subdivides the extent of epiphyseal involvement into four groups. Group 1 (25%) and 2 (50%) have partial head involvement with a clear demarcation between involved and uninvolved tissues; group 3

None of the authors received financial support for this study.

a Université de Montpellier, Faculté de Médecine, 2, rue de l'Ecole de Médecine 34000, Montpellier, France
b Service de Chirurgie Infantile, Centre Hospitalier Universitaire Estaing, 1, place Lucie Aubrac, 63004, Clermont Ferrand, France
* Corresponding author.
E-mail address: canavese_federico@yahoo.fr

Orthop Clin N Am 42 (2011) 297–302
doi:10.1016/j.ocl.2011.04.003

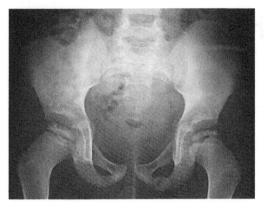

Fig. 1. Plain radiography. It is best to initiate imaging of LCP disease with anteroposterior (AP) and frog lateral plain radiographs, and to image both hips to eliminate contralateral disease. AP radiograph shows a boy with bilateral disease.

and 4 are severe forms and the extent of femoral head involvement is sub-total (75%) and total (100%), respectively. Catterall showed that the prognosis is proportional to the degree of radiological involvement and groups can be recognised in the early stages and do not change during the course of the disease.[6–8,13]

Salter and Thompson classification (1983)
According to the extent of the subchondral crescentic line initially described by Waldenstrom in 1938, Salter and Thompson established a radiographic classification. In type-A, the extent of the subchondral fracture is less than 50% of the femoral head, and in type-B it is over 50%. Salter and Thompson found the subchondral fracture in only 23% of the children who were initially studied and that its duration varied directly with the age of the patient at the onset of the disease, ranging from an average of 3 months when the patient's age at onset was 4 years or less, to an average of 8.5 months when the onset was at the age of 10 years or more.[9,13,14]

Herring classification (1992)
Herring and colleagues introduced the lateral pillar classification which is based on radiolucency the femoral head's lateral pillar during fragmentation. This classification system is widely used and degree of involvement is assessed on AP radiographs of the hip. According to the extent of lateral pillar involvement, four groups can be identified: A, B, B/C border and C. In group A, the lateral pillar is radiographically normal whereas in group C less that 50% remains visible. Herring's classsification may help in determining the prognosis but can only applied after the disease has progressed to the stage of fragmentation.[10,13,15]

Plain radiographs can also be used to assess femoral head shape at skeletal maturity. Two radiologic classifications are possible.

Mose classification (1980)
A radiolucent template, with concentric circles, is placed over the femoral head on AP and lateral radiographs. If the femoral head spheroid does not deviate more that 1 mm from the template, the result is considered as good. On the other hand, femoral heads deviating within 2 mm or more than 3 mm from the template are considered to be fair and poor, respectively.

According to Mose,[18] measurements should be made no earlier than age 16 years, when growth has stopped and femoral head shape no longer changes.

Stulberg classification (1981)
Stulberg and colleagues[19] developed a 5-group classification system that correlated radiographic appearance of the femoral head and the acetabulum at skeletal maturity with the long-term degenerative arthritis. Hips of classes 1 and 2 are spherically congruent, have a good long-term prognosis, and correspond to Mose's good and fair results. Hips of classes 3 and 4 are aspherically congruent, have intermediate prognosis, and correspond to Mose's poor results. Hips of class 5 are completely aspherical and incongruent, and are at high risk of early degenerative joint disease.

Neyt and colleagues[20] suggested that the Stulberg classification is not a highly reliable tool for the evaluation of the radiographs of patients who are managed for LCP disease at or after skeletal maturity. It was therefore proposed that hips could be divided into spherical (Stulberg 1 and 2) and nonspherical (Stulberg 3–5) only.

Bone Scintigraphy

Conway classification (1993)
Conway[21] described a scintigraphic classification system with prognostic significance, which precedes radiographic changes by an average of 3 months. This classification does not describe the extent of femoral head involvement, rather the scintigraphic patterns associated with the revascularization versus recanalization process.

Conway's scintigraphic classification identifies types A ('all right'), B ('bad'), and C ('regression') pathways. The type-A pathway is characterized by early appearance of a lateral column formation in the capital femoral epiphysis, indicating early and rapid revascularization. The type-B pathway is characterized by centrally located scintigraphic activity arising from the base of the femoral epiphysis or by the absence of radioactivity in the

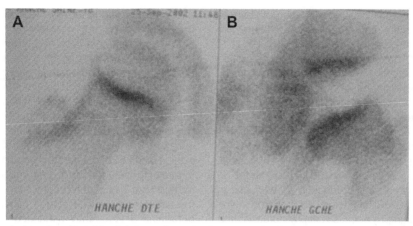

Fig. 2. Bone scintigraphy of left hip. (*A*) Contralateral side is normal. (*B*) A type B pathway characterized by centrally located scintigraphic activity arising from the base of the femoral epiphysis.

epiphysis after 5 months (**Fig. 2**). The type-C pathway indicates is a regression from pathway A to B, but is very rare.[5,21–23]

Van Campenhout and colleagues[22] found a significant correlation between vascularization pattern and the radiographic classification of Herring and Catterall,[6–8,10,15] and recommended including serial scintigraphy in the early evaluation of the patient who has LCP disease. Comte and colleagues[12] and Oufroukhi and colleagues[23] confirmed the high prognostic value of bone scanning in LCP disease: if a type-B pathway is identified, the child has a higher risk for poor prognosis. A hip presenting with a type-A pathway is most likely to show a Catterall 1-2 or Herring A-B subgroup, as the lateral column is already present before radiologic changes occur. On the other hand, a hip presenting with a type-B or type-C pathway is most likely to show a Catterall 3-4 or Herring B/C border-C subgroup, with lateral column completely absent. Two bone scans are necessary: one is performed at diagnosis and the second one at 4 to 5 months. When serial scintigraphy is included in the early evaluation of patients with LCP disease, earlier diagnosis and prognosis may lead to earlier containment and, eventually, better outcome.

Magnetic Resonance Imaging

Magnetic resonance imaging (MRI) with conventional sequencing has been proved to be sensitive in the diagnosis of LCP disease, and may be used to assess the extent of femoral head infarction. Overall, MRI scans provide a good anatomic picture of the cartilaginous femoral head including flat or round shape, the degree of extrusion of the femoral head, the degree of superolateral displacement of the femoral head (subluxation), the eversion of the labrum, and the extent of necrosis.

However, it is not accurate enough to describe the stages of healing, and in the early stages of the disease may sometimes fail to depict epiphyseal ischemia.[24–27] Sales de Gauzy and colleagues[28] evaluated hip subluxation in LCP disease, comparing MRI with plain radiographs. Using plain radiographs, they measured the percentage of the bony femoral head that was uncovered beneath the bony acetabulum; however, using MRI they measured the percentage of the cartilaginous femoral head that was uncovered by the cartilaginous acetabulum. Approximately one-third of the patients studied were well contained on the plain radiographs but were subluxated on the MRI, due to thickening of the cartilaginous portion of the femoral head. In virtually all affected hips the MRI images can identify the subchondral fracture as a low-intensity zone in the subchondral region that persists well beyond the early phase of the disease.[9,25,26]

Healing can also be assessed with imaging. MRI shows healing as an increase in normal signal intensity. When repair takes place, the fibrous repair tissue is shown on the T1-weighted images as a semi-lunar, cup-shaped, low-intensity band. The outer zone of the repair tissue is of low intensity in both T1-weighted and T2-weighted images, demarcating living bone from necrotic bone.[24–26]

For serial follow-up and to assess the extent of healing of the femoral head, plain radiographs are usually done as well as MRI.[27]

When progressive subluxation of the femoral head is suspected, MRI may be performed instead of arthrography. This imaging may help avoid arthrography, an invasive procedure that often requires general anesthesia.

The main advantage of MRI is that is a nonionizing examination that provides good anatomic images. The downsides of MRI are cost, availability, and the need for sedation of younger children because of the requirement of immobility during examination.

Dynamic gadolinium-enhanced subtraction (DGS) MRI allows early detection of epiphyseal ischemia and different revascularization patterns, as described by Sebag and colleagues.[29] Lamer and colleagues[30] showed that there is total agreement between DGS MRI and bone scintigraphy, and stated that DGS MRI may be used as a possible nonionizing substitute for bone scintigraphy, as all scintigraphic uptakes could be demonstrated on DGS MRI. Lamer and colleagues showed that in particular, DGS MRI has reperfusion patterns similar to bone scintigraphy because of early increased and persisting enhancement within the revascularized zones as compared with normal hip enhancement. The increased gadolinium uptake is probably related to increased vascularity, vasodilatation, greater capillary permeability, and diffusion in the reparative process. Moreover, MRI provides optimal anatomic detail compared with scintigraphy.[24,29]

Merlini and colleagues[31] have more recently compared diffusion-weighted imaging findings (DWI MRI) with DGS MRI, and have preliminarily concluded that DWI MRI is a noninvasive method that can help to distinguish between LCP disease with favorable and unfavorable prognosis.

Arthrography

Arthrography may be used to evaluate possible methods of treatment. Arthrography should be performed in the operating room under strict sterile conditions and technique. It is rarely useful in the earliest stage of the disease, because arthrographic findings may be normal or show just a subtle flattening of the femoral head.[32–34]

Although MRI can also demonstrate cartilage surfaces and bony articular structures, arthrography offers the opportunity to evaluate coverage and mobility under direct vision during fluoroscopy (**Fig. 3**). In particular, when severe collapse and flattening of the femoral head is present, arthrography is helpful in assessing containability before any treatment is started. Arthrography can help identify the best position for femoral head containment and demonstrate absence of hinge abduction prior to containment surgery. Jaramillo and colleagues[35] found that multipositional MRI with open magnet was comparable with arthrography for demonstrating containment and congruency of the articular surfaces of the hip. However, in the evaluation of deformity or loss of the spherical nature of the femoral head, open-magnet MRI performed less well. Arthrography may also be performed during the late stages of remodeling to determine if apparently nonunited fragments of bone are free or covered by cartilage.

Laredo classification (1992)

Laredo established an arthrographic classification that identifies 5 types of hip essentially based on femoral head shape and position of the labrum.

Type 1 hips are normal. In type 2 hips, the femoral head is still spherical but is larger than normal, whereas in type 3 the femoral head is ovoid in shape. Type 4 hips have a large and flattened femoral head, and the labrum loses its concavity and becomes elevated and straightened. Moreover, hinge abduction is present. Type 5 hips show a femoral head larger than normal and saddle shaped; the labrum is still elevated and can sometimes be everted. All hips, from type 2 to type 5, show femoral head extrusion at neutral position and normal coverage at about 30° of abduction with slight internal rotation.[32–34]

Computed Tomography

Computed tomography (CT) scans allow early diagnosis of bone collapse, curvilinear zones of sclerosis, and subtle changes in the bone trabecular pattern. CT scans can also identify intraosseous cysts in later stages of LCP disease. Moreover, CT provides precise information about

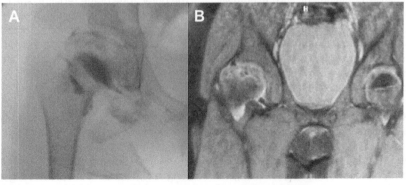

Fig. 3. (*A*) Arthrography and (*B*) magnetic resonance imaging of the right hip.

the anatomic relationship between femoral head and acetabulum, and allows study of the 3-dimensional nature of the femoral head deformity. However, its use is limited by the comparatively high radiation dose.[1,36]

Ultrasonography

Ultrasonography takes a few minutes, does not irradiate the patient, and can be performed with relatively inexpensive equipment. It usually shows effusion in the hip which, especially when persistent, should raise the suspicion of early LCP disease. However, ultrasonography is nonspecific and primarily helps to provide clues to differentiate early LCP disease from transient synovitis of the hip. In patients with transient synovitis, capsular distension is attributed to synovial effusion, whereas in patients with LCP disease it is usually produced by thickening of the synovial membrane. Moreover, ultrasonography can provide some clues about coverage, flattening of the femoral head, and irregularity or deformation of the bony epiphysis.[37,38]

SUMMARY

Several imaging techniques are possible and available. Nevertheless, not all examinations can be performed at the same time and with the same results. The imaging technique of choice should take into account the clinical examination of the patient, and both the severity and the stage of the disease.

1. Physis involvement has a high predictive value in LCP disease, but the extent of bone necrosis is probably the main risk factor influencing prognosis ("surgery proposes, the growth cartilage decides").
2. Plain radiographs and clinical examination are the first step toward diagnosis and assessment of the disease.
3. Scintigraphy allows early detection of severe forms, so that earlier containment may positively influence outcome.
4. MRI has gained an important place in the evaluation of the severity of the disease. Anatomic changes induced by the disease can be evaluated with precision.
5. Dynamic arthrography helps decide whether containment is possible and to select the best surgical option for containment of the affected hip.
6. CT images provide precise information on the relationship between femoral head and acetabulum, and allow study of the 3-dimensional nature of the deformity.

7. For those children with bone age of 6 years or more, early detection of severe forms may improve prognosis.

REFERENCES

1. Jaramillo D. What is the optimal imaging of osteonecrosis, Perthes, and bone infarcts? Pediatr Radiol 2009;39(S2):S216–9.
2. Hubbard AM, Dormans JP. Evaluation of developmental dysplasia, Perthes disease, and neuromuscular dysplasia of the hip in children before and after surgery: an imaging update. AJR Am J Roentgenol 1995;164:1067–73.
3. Klisic P. Perthes' disease. Int Orthop 1984;8:95–102.
4. Kaniklides C, Lonnerholm T, Moberg A, et al. Legg Perthes Calvé disease. Comparison of conventional radiography, MR imaging, bone scintigraphy and arthrography. Acta Radiol 1995;36:434–9.
5. Canavese F, Dimeglio A. Legg-Perthes-Calvé disease: prognostic results in children under six years old. J Bone Joint Surg Br 2008;90:940–5.
6. Catterall A. Legg-Perthes-Calvé disease. Edinburgh (United Kingdom): Churchill Livingstone; 1982.
7. Catterall A. The natural history of Perthes' disease. J Bone Joint Surg Br 1971;53:37–53.
8. Catterall A. Natural history, classification, and x-ray signs in Legg-Calvé-Perthes' disease. Acta Orthop Belg 1980;46:346–51.
9. Salter RB, Thompson GH. Legg-Calvé-Perthes disease. The prognostic significance of the subchondral fracture and a two-group classification of the femoral head involvement. J Bone Joint Surg Am 1984;66:479–89.
10. Herring JA, Neustadt JB, Williams JJ, et al. The lateral pillar classification of Legg-Calvé-Perthes disease. J Pediatr Orthop 1992;12:143–50.
11. Tsao AK, Dias LS, Conway JJ, et al. The prognostic value and significance of serial bone scintigraphy in Legg-Calvé-Perthes disease. J Pediatr Orthop 1997;17:230–9.
12. Comte F, De Rosa V, Zekri H, et al. Confirmation of the early prognostic value of bone scanning and pinhole imaging of the hip in Legg-Calvé-Perthes disease. J Nucl Med 2003;44(11):1761–6.
13. Wiig O, Svenningsen S, Terjesen T. Evaluation of the subchondral fracture in predicting the extent of femoral head necrosis in Perthes disease: a prospective study of 92 patients. J Pediatr Orthop B 2004;13:293–8.
14. Wiig O, Terjesen T, Svenningsen S. Inter-observer reliability of radiographic classifications and measurements in the assessment of Perthes' disease. Acta Orthop Scand 2002;73:523–30.
15. Herring JA, Kim HT, Browne RH. Legg-Calvé-Perthes disease. Part I: classification of radiographs with use

of the modified lateral pillar and Stulberg classifications. J Bone Joint Surg Am 2004;86:2103–20.

16. Lappin K, Kealey D, Cosgrove A. Herring classification: how useful is the initial radiograph? J Pediatr Orthop 2002;22:479–82.

17. Price CT. The lateral pillar classification for Legg-Calvé-Perthes disease. J Pediatr Orthop 2007;27:592–3.

18. Mose K. Methods of measuring Legg-Calvé-Perthes disease with special regard to the prognosis. Clin Orthop 1980;150:103–9.

19. Stulberg SD, Cooperman DR, Wallensten R. The natural history of Legg-Calvé-Perthes disease. J Bone Joint Surg Am 1981;63:1095–108.

20. Neyt JG, Weinstein SL, Spratt KF, et al. Stulberg classification system for evaluation of Legg-Calvé-Perthes disease: intra-rater and inter-rater reliability. J Bone Joint Surg Am 1999;81:1209–16.

21. Conway JJ. A scintigraphic classification of Legg-Perthes-Calvé disease. Semin Nucl Med 1993;23:274–95.

22. Van Campenhout A, Moens P, Fabry G. Serial bone scintigraphy in Legg–Calvé-Perthes disease: correlation with the Catterall and Herring classification. J Pediatr Orthop B 2006;15:6–10.

23. Oufroukhi Y, Biyi A, Doudouh A. Intérêt de l'utilisation de la scintigraphie osseuse dans le diagnostic et le suivi de l'ostéochondrite primitive de la hanche. Médecine Nucléaire 2009;33:211–5.

24. Scoles PV, Yoon YS, Makley JT, et al. Nuclear magnetic resonance imaging in Legg-Calvé-Perthes disease. J Bone Joint Surg Am 1984;66:1357–63.

25. de Sanctis N, Rega AN, Rondinella F. Prognostic evaluation of Legg-Calvé-Perthes disease by MRI. Part I: the role of physeal involvement. J Pediatr Orthop 2000;20:455–62.

26. de Sanctis N, Rondinella F. Prognostic evaluation of Legg-Calvé-Perthes disease by MRI. Part II: pathomorphogenesis and new classification. J Pediatr Orthop 2000;20:463–70.

27. Hochbergs P, Eckerwall G, Egund N, et al. Femoral head shape in Legg Perthes Calvé disease. Correlation between conventional radiology, arthrography and MR imaging. Acta Radiol 1994;35:545–8.

28. Sales de Gauzy J, Kerdiles N, Baunin C, et al. Imaging evaluation of subluxation in Legg-Calvé-Perthes' disease: magnetic resonance imaging compared with the plain radiograph. J Pediatr Orthop 1997;6:235–8.

29. Sebag G, Ducou Le Pointe H, Klein I, et al. Dynamic gadolinium-enhanced subtraction MR imaging: a simple technique for early diagnosis of Legg-Perthes-Calvé disease: preliminary results. Pediatr Radiol 1997;27:216–20.

30. Lamer S, Dorgeret S, Khairouni A, et al. Femoral head vascularisation in Legg-Calvé-Perthes disease: comparison of dynamic gadolinium-enhanced subtraction MRI with bone scintigraphy. Pediatr Radiol 2002;32:580–5.

31. Merlini L, Combescure C, De Rosa V, et al. Diffusion-weighted imaging findings in Perthes disease with dynamic gadolinium-enhanced subtracted (DGS) MR correlation: a preliminary study. Pediatr Radiol 2010;40:318–25.

32. Kamegaya M, Moriya H, Tsuchiya K, et al. Arthrography of early Perthes' disease. Swelling of the ligamentum teres as a cause of subluxation. J Bone Joint Surg Br 1989;71:413–7.

33. Laredo FJ. Legg-Perthes-Calvé disease: arthrographic classification. Rev Bras Ortop 1992;27:7–10 [in Portuguese].

34. Milani C, Laredo Filho J, Ishida A, et al. [Technique of interpretation of the images of the femoral head obtained by arthrography and MRI in Legg-Perthes-Calvé disease: study of 60 patients]. Revista Brasileira de Ortopedia Pediatrica 2000;1:6–14 [in Portuguese].

35. Jaramillo D, Galen TA, Winalski CS. Legg-Perthes-Calvé disease: MR imaging evaluation during manual positioning of the hip: comparison with conventional arthrography. Radiology 1999;12:519–25.

36. Shingade VU, Song HR, Lee SH, et al. The sagging rope sign in achondroplasia: different from Perthes' disease. Skeletal Radiol 2006;35:923–8.

37. Futami T, Kasahara Y, Suzuki S, et al. Ultrasonography in transient synovitis and early Perthes' disease. J Bone Joint Surg Br 1991;73:635–9.

38. Suzuki S, Awaya G, Okada Y, et al. Examination by ultrasound of Legg-Calvé-Perthes disease. Clin Orthop Relat Res 1987;220:130–6.

Prognostic Factors and Outcome Measures in Perthes Disease

Benjamin Joseph, MS Orth, MCh Orth

KEYWORDS

- Perthes disease • Prognostic variables
- Outcome measures • Treatment planning

The term "prognosis" is derived from the Greek word *prognostikos*, which means "of knowledge beforehand." It is worthwhile keeping this interpretation of the term in mind while considering various factors that influence the prognosis in Perthes disease.

As in the case of any disease, the importance of identifying reliable prognostic factors in Perthes disease is to enable the clinician to institute appropriate intervention to minimize the risk of an unsatisfactory outcome. Thus, the value of a particular prognostic indicator depends on 3 factors:

1. Can the prognostic factor be reproducibly and consistently identified?
2. Does the prognostic factor reliably predict a potentially adverse outcome?
3. Can the prognostic factor be recognized sufficiently early in the course of the disease for any intervention to be effective in preventing the adverse outcome?

In the ensuing discussion an attempt is made to evaluate various prognostic factors in the light of these 3 characteristics.

OUTCOMES IN PERTHES DISEASE

A large proportion of children who develop Perthes disease will end up with normal or near-normal hips that function well throughout their lives; this would be an optimal outcome.[1,2] However, some children will go on to develop secondary degenerative arthritis in adult life.[3–6] Thus, the poor outcome of Perthes disease is development of secondary degenerative arthritis of the hip in early or mid adult life, and treatment in childhood is aimed at preventing this.

Although the final outcome should be assessed in adult life, the interim outcome of Perthes disease may be assessed at two points in childhood and adolescence; the first is when the disease heals and the second is at skeletal maturity. A suboptimal outcome at either of these two points will have a direct bearing on the third and final outcome in adult life.

First Level of Outcome

Suboptimal outcomes at healing

1. The femoral head may lose it spherical shape and become
   a. Ovoid (**Fig. 1**A)
   b. Frankly irregular in contour (**Fig. 1**B)
2. The femoral head may become enlarged
   a. The acetabulum may also enlarge proportionately to cover the femoral head
   b. The femoral head may be too large to be covered by the acetabulum (**Fig. 1**C)
3. The femoral head and the acetabulum may no longer be congruous.

Second Level of Outcome

Suboptimal outcome at skeletal maturity

1. The femoral neck may be foreshortened on account of growth inhibition of the capital

The author has nothing to disclose.
Paediatric Orthopaedic Service, Department of Orthopaedics, Kasturba Medical College, Madhavnagar, Manipal 576 104, Karnataka State, India
E-mail address: bjosephortho@yahoo.co.in

Orthop Clin N Am 42 (2011) 303–315
doi:10.1016/j.ocl.2011.03.004
0030-5898/11/$ – see front matter © 2011 Elsevier Inc. All rights reserved.

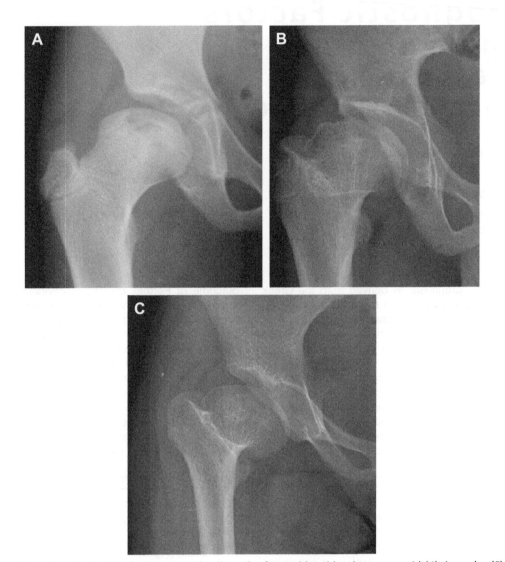

Fig. 1. Examples of suboptimal outcomes at healing. The femoral head has become ovoid (*A*), irregular (*B*), or enlarged (*C*) in these hips when the disease has healed.

femoral growth plate with associated "over-growth" of the greater trochanter (**Fig. 2**). Although there may be a suggestion of this when the disease heals, the full extent of the growth abnormality will not be evident until complete cessation of skeletal growth has taken place.

2. Any of the 3 suboptimal outcomes if noted at healing will be evident at skeletal maturity (see **Fig. 2**), though some minor change may have occurred between healing and skeletal maturity as a consequence of remodeling.

Third Level of Outcome: Long-Term Outcome

Suboptimal outcome in adult life

Degenerative arthritis of the hip

All of the suboptimal outcomes noted at skeletal maturity will be evident in the adult. However, they are inconsequential if the patient has no symptoms or if there is no evidence of arthritis.

The outcomes at healing, skeletal maturity, and in the adult may be termed the short-term outcome, the intermediate-term outcome, and the long-term outcome, respectively.

OUTCOME MEASURES
Short-Term Outcome (At Healing)

Assessment of the shape of the femoral head

The most widely used method of assessment of sphericity of the femoral head is that described by Mose and colleagues.[6,7] Mose used a transparent template of concentric circles 2 mm apart

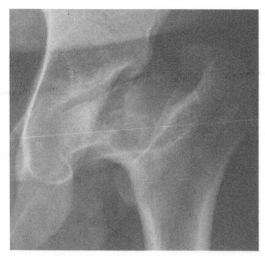

Fig. 2. Appearance of the hip of a patient with healed Perthes disease at skeletal maturity showing suboptimal outcomes. The femoral head is not spherical, its contour is irregular, and the femoral neck is short. The full extent of trochanteric "overgrowth" is evident now.

to place over the radiograph so as to overlay the femoral head (**Fig. 3**A).

The head is considered to be spherical when the articular margin of the femoral head perfectly matches the arc of a circle of the same radius on both the anteroposterior and lateral radiographs. The head is regarded as ovoid if the femoral articular margin fits the arc of a circle perfectly in both views but the radius of the femoral head differs on the anteroposterior and lateral views by 2 mm or less. The head is regarded as being flattened or irregular if the articular margin of the femoral head does not conform to the arc of a circle in either view, or if the articular surface conforms to the arcs of circles in both views, but the radius of the femoral head differs in the two views by more than 2 mm.

Practical problems that have been reported with the use of the Mose template are difficulty in visualizing the margin of the femoral head through the template and identifying with certainty the circle that matches the articular margins in the anteroposterior and lateral radiographs.[8] Because the circles are so close together (2 mm), parallax errors may also occur. Herring and colleagues[8] suggested a method using a compass and a protractor to locate the center of the femoral head and then marking the best-fit circle to match the radius of the femoral head. Edgren[9] used a series of transparent plastic circles of various sizes instead of a single template. The author has been using a similar set of translucent plastic disks of varying diameters (see **Fig. 3**B) for several

years. The disk that best fits the contour of the femoral head is selected, as shown in **Fig. 3**. This method is a lot easier than using the original Mose template and the method described by Herring.

The contour of the femoral head can also be assessed by digitizing the tracings of radiographs and matching them to a best-fit circle with the help of a computer.[10] With more centers using Picture Archiving and Communication Systems (PACS) and viewing radiographs on computer screens, the template itself may be used less frequently, but exactly the same measurements can easily be made with software programs designed for radiographic measurements.

Assessment of the size of the femoral head

The Mose template, translucent disks as described earlier, or software programs may be used to accurately measure the radius of the femoral head. The radius of the femoral head of the affected side is compared with that of the unaffected hip to estimate the degree of enlargement of the head in unilateral cases. Accurate estimates of the size of the femoral head may be impossible if the femoral head is grossly deformed, as in **Fig. 2**.

Assessment of femoral head coverage by the acetabulum

The center-edge (CE) angle of Wiberg[11] and the acetabular-head index (AHI) are methods for estimating the extent to which the acetabulum covers the femoral head. The Reimer migration index,[12] on the other hand, measures the extent of the femoral head that is uncovered (**Fig. 4**).

If the femoral head is distorted it may be difficult or impossible to accurately locate the center of the femoral head, and in such instances the CE angle cannot be reliably estimated; the AHI and the migration index are not influenced by the shape of the femoral head. The author prefers to use the Reimer migration index, as it is included in commercially available software programs for making measurements on hip radiographs.

Assessment of the femoral head shape and congruency of the hip

In 1981 Stulberg and colleagues[3] suggested a classification that has since been widely used to describe the outcome of Perthes disease. The affected hip can be classified into 1 of 5 classes (Class I to Class V) from plain radiographs in this system at healing, at skeletal maturity, or in the adult. The classification system takes into consideration the shape and size of the femoral head and neck, the shape of the acetabulum, and the congruence of the femoral head and the acetabulum. Class I hips are essentially normal while all

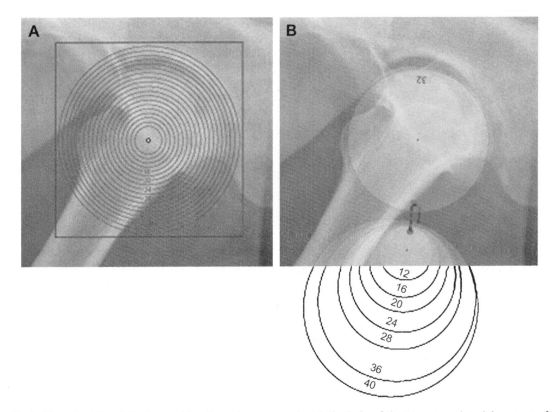

Fig. 3. The sphericity of the femoral head may be measured with the help of the Mose template (*A*) or a set of translucent disks of varying radii (*B*).

other Classes show varying degrees of abnormality (**Table 1**).

Although the classification system was described in 1981 its reproducibility was only assessed 18 years later by Neyt and colleagues,[13] who suggested that the reproducibility of the classification system is not very good. Herring and colleagues[8] more recently suggested some modifications in the classification system to improve the reproducibility; in particular, they recommended actually drawing the best-fit circle to assess the shape of the femoral head. Herring and colleagues noted excellent reproducibility of the Stulberg classification with these modifications, with weighted kappa values of 0.82[8]; an identical kappa value was reported by Shah and

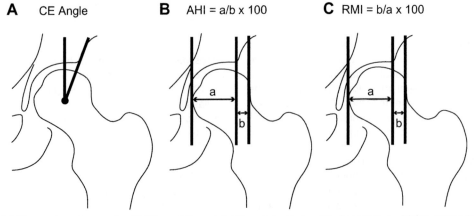

Fig. 4. (*A*) The center-edge angle of Wiberg (CE angle), (*B*) acetabular-head index (AHI), and (*C*) Reimer migration index (RMI).

Table 1
Stulberg classification of outcome of Perthes disease

Class	Femoral Head Shape	Femoral Head Size, Femoral Neck Length, and Configuration of the Acetabulum	Congruency
Class I	Spherical	Normal size of femoral head, neck, and acetabulum	Congruous (spherical congruency)
Class II	Spherical	Coxa magna, coxa brevis, or acetabular dysplasia present	Congruous (spherical congruency)
Class III	Ovoid	Coxa magna, coxa brevis, or acetabular dysplasia present	Congruous (aspherical congruency)
Class IV	Flat (irregular)	Coxa magna, coxa brevis, or acetabular dysplasia present	Congruous (aspherical congruency)
Class V	Flat (irregular)	Mild or no coxa magna, no coxa brevis, normal-shaped acetabulum, and no acetabular dysplasia	Incongruous (aspherical incongruency)

Data from Stulberg SD, Cooperman DR, Wallensten R. The natural history of Legg-Calvé-Perthes disease. J Bone Joint Surg Am 1981;63(7):1095–108.

colleagues,[14] who also used templates to measure the sphericity of the femoral head while applying the Stulberg classification.

Wiig and colleagues[15] combined Stulberg Classes I and II into one group and similarly combined Stulberg Classes IV and V. These investigators reported satisfactory reproducibility of the 3-group Stulberg classification, with a kappa value of 0.70.

One of the limitations of the Stulberg classification is that it is a discrete ordinal scale, and if this outcome measure is used in long-term prospective studies the sample size has to be a great deal larger than when an outcome measure with a continuous scale is used. For this reason the deformity index, a continuous measure proposed by Nelson and colleagues,[16] is an attractive option. Nelson and colleagues demonstrated that the reproducibility of estimation of this index that measures changes in the epiphyseal height and width is excellent.

Intermediate-Term Outcome (at Skeletal Maturity)

Assessment of the shape and size of the femoral head, and the extent of femoral head coverage
These variables can be assessed as done at healing.

Assessment of the level of the trochanter in relation to the femoral head
The articulo-trochanteric distance initially described by Edgren[9] and the center-trochanteric distance (**Fig. 5**) measured on anteroposterior radiographs of the pelvis assess the extent of

greater trochanteric "overgrowth" that has occurred on account of growth inhibition of the femoral capital physis.[17,18] The latter measurement cannot be used if the femoral head is distorted, as the center of the femoral head cannot be accurately located.

Assessment of limb length
Clinical or radiographic measurement of the limb lengths will help to quantify limb length inequality.

Clinical assessment of hip function
Any of the standard scoring systems that evaluate hip function may be employed.[19,20]

In Adult Life

In addition to all the assessments performed at skeletal maturity, radiological evaluation to identify signs of arthritic change is essential.

PROGNOSTIC FACTORS THAT MAY PREDICT OUTCOMES
Clinical Factors

Age at the onset of the disease
There appears be universal agreement that the younger the child at onset of Perthes, the better the prognosis.[1,4,21–24]

Though children younger than 5 years generally have the best prognosis, not all children under 5 have a good outcome (**Fig. 6**).[25–27] Fabry and colleagues[25] reviewed a series of 30 patients who were younger than 5 years at the onset of symptoms. At skeletal maturity 41.6% had nonspherical femoral heads and a third of the children had incongruous hips. This result clearly suggests that while age is undoubtedly an

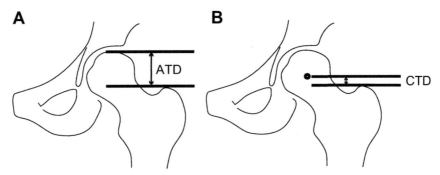

Fig. 5. The extent of relative trochanteric overgrowth may be estimated by measuring the articulo-trochanteric distance (ATD) (*A*) or the center-trochanteric distance (CTD) (*B*).

important prognostic indicator, other factors must influence the outcome.

The prognosis does get poorer as the age at onset of the disease increases, and outcome is uniformly dismal when the onset of the disease is in adolescence.[28–31]

Gender

Some investigators had suggested that the prognosis is worse in girls than in boys, and it was assumed that this was on account of girls reaching skeletal maturity earlier than boys, leaving less time for remodeling of the femoral head between healing of the disease and skeletal maturity.[21,32]

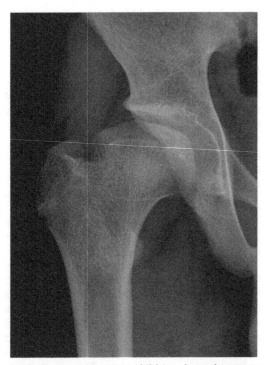

Fig. 6. Poor outcome in a child in whom the age at onset of Perthes disease was younger than 5 years.

However, there is no strong evidence to suggest that the prognosis is indeed worse in girls than in boys.[33]

Factors Identified on Plain Radiographs

Extent of epiphyseal involvement

Catterall,[34] in a landmark article, classified the extent of epiphyseal involvement into 4 groups ranging from involvement of only the anterolateral aspect of the epiphysis (Group I) to total epiphyseal involvement (Group IV). He also showed that the prognosis is poorest in Group IV disease and best in Group I. The impression that the greater the extent of epiphyseal infarction, the poorer the prognosis has been supported by several subsequent reports.[21,35–37]

A major shortcoming of the Catterall classification is that the disease has to evolve to the stage of fragmentation before the hip can be classified into one of Catterall's groups, and this is one of the drawbacks of using this classification for treatment planning. The reproducibility of the system is also not excellent, particularly in distinguishing between Group II and Group III involvement.[38,39]

Salter and Thompson[40] demonstrated that the extent of epiphyseal infarction can be determined very early in the course of the disease by noting the length of the subchondral fracture line that may be identified in the early stage of avascular necrosis (**Fig. 7**). Their two-group classification is easy to apply, but the shortcoming is that the subchondral fracture line is only visible in approximately one-third of children with Perthes disease.[41,42]

Extent of epiphyseal collapse

For several years investigators have appreciated the fact that the extent of collapse of the capital femoral epiphysis reflects the severity of Perthes disease. In 1936 Eyre-Brook[43] described the epiphyseal index, and in 1942 Sjovall[44] described the epiphyseal quotient to measure the extent of collapse of the epiphysis. These indices were

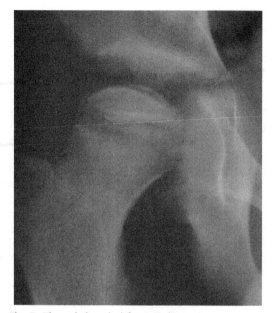

Fig. 7. The subchondral fracture line.

greater the collapse of the lateral pillar of the epiphysis, the poorer the prognosis.[49–53]

The major drawback of using this classification as a guide to treatment is that the collapse of the lateral pillar can only be determined during the fragmentation stage; the more severe cases will progressively collapse while under observation. Thus, the degree of collapse may increase as the disease passes from the early stage of fragmentation to the late part of the stage of fragmentation, making it difficult to allocate the hip to a specific class or to guide treatment (**Fig. 8**).[54]

Metaphyseal abnormalities

Diffuse metaphyseal osteoporosis, metaphyseal cysts, and widening of the femoral metaphysis have been identified as poor prognostic indicators.[55–57] These metaphyseal changes usually develop in the stage of fragmentation and are seldom encountered in the stage of avascular necrosis.[58]

also often used as outcome measures, but they were limited to evaluation of only the short-term outcome or up until closure of the physis.[43,45–47]

Herring and colleagues[48] introduced a classification of the extent of epiphyseal collapse during the stage of fragmentation with specific reference to the lateral part of the epiphysis, which they named the "lateral pillar." The prognostic significance of this classification was emphasized by these investigators, and several others have subsequently endorsed the impression that the

Acetabular abnormalities

Altered contour of the acetabulum, referred to as bicompartmentalization, has also been associated with a poor outcome (**Fig. 9**).[59] Whenever bicompartmentalization occurs, the femoral head articulates with the lateral part of the acetabulum and consequently the lateral part of the femoral head extrudes outside the confines of the acetabulum. This and other acetabular changes that are associated with a poor outcome again usually only develop during the stage of fragmentation.[58,59]

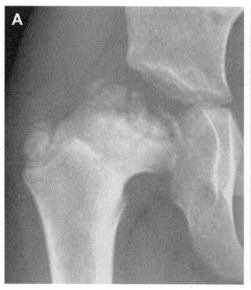
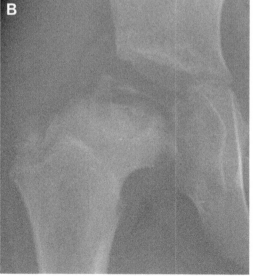

Fig. 8. (A, B) The extent of epiphyseal collapse may increase as the disease progresses. The height of the lateral pillar has decreased in this child.

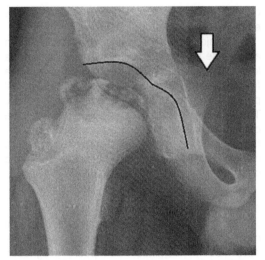

Fig. 9. Acetabular changes in a child with Perthes disease include bicompartmentalization (*line*) and ischium varum (*arrow*).

Catterall's "head-at-risk" signs

Catterall defined some radiological signs that were of prognostic significance,[34] which included diffuse metaphyseal reaction, calcification lateral to the epiphysis, Gage's sign (**Fig. 10**), horizontal alignment of the femoral capital physis, and epiphyseal extrusion. Whereas some investigators have suggested that these are good prognostic indicators, others have questioned the efficacy of these signs.[60] In particular, Loder demonstrated that there was no difference between the physeal inclination in the contralateral normal hips and affected hips in 40 children with unilateral Perthes disease.[61]

Calcification lateral to the epiphysis also cannot be regarded as a "head-at-risk" sign, as it indicates that the disease has progressed beyond the stage of fragmentation and signifies displacement of an already flattened or deformed epiphysis.[60]

Extent of epiphyseal extrusion

Of all the prognostic factors that have been identified, epiphyseal extrusion is by far the most important. Extrusion of the lateral part of the epiphysis outside the confines of the acetabulum has also been referred to as "loss of containment" and "lateral subluxation." Studies have shown that extrusion predisposes to femoral head deformation,[62–64] and it has also been shown that when more than 20% of the width of the femoral head extrudes there is a high chance of the femoral head becoming deformed (**Fig. 11**).[65] A study on the natural history of the disease has shown that extrusion often commences early in the course of the disease and progresses as the disease evolves.[58] Extrusion tends to be more pronounced in the older child, and when there is extensive involvement of the epiphysis.

Among all the prognostic factors that have been identified, epiphyseal extrusion is the only factor that can be modified by treatment. Treatment by containment methods attempts to either preempt or reverse extrusion.

Factors Noted on Arthrograms, Magnetic Resonance Images, and Isotope Bone Scans

Although most prognostic indicators described in the literature are based on plain radiographic

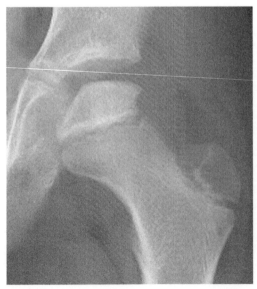

Fig. 10. Gage's sign: a triangular lucent area on the lateral aspect of the epiphysis.

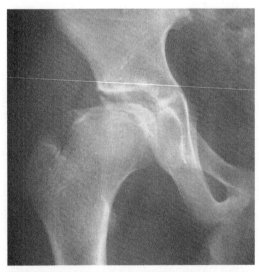

Fig. 11. Femoral head deformation has occurred in a child in whom femoral head extrusion exceeded 20%.

appearances, a few investigators have identified prognostic factors on arthrograms and magnetic resonance imaging (MRI) scans.

The extent of epiphyseal infarction, involvement of the physis, and the extent of epiphyseal extrusion detected on the MRI were shown to have prognostic significance.[66,67] One of the advantages of MRI is that physeal involvement, which cannot be demonstrated by other imaging methods, can be identified on the MRI scan. The estimate of the extent of femoral head extrusion on the MRI scan is also more precise than that made on plain radiographs, as the cartilaginous components of the femoral head and acetabulum can be visualized on MRI.

Some surgeons advocate the routine use of arthrograms to delineate the contour of the femoral head, and suggest that arthrography in the stages of fragmentation or early reconstitution can reliably predict the shape of the femoral head at skeletal maturity.[49,68,69]

One of the problems with the routine use of arthrograms and MRI scans to prognosticate outcome is deciding on the optimal time to perform the scan. Because various prognostic factors manifest at different times during the course of the disease, a scan or arthrogram done at a particular point of time may not demonstrate the critical features. The use of sequential arthrograms is not justified because it is an invasive procedure, and repeated MRI scans may be limited by cost factors.

Conway[70] identified two distinct patterns of revascularization of the femoral epiphysis on isotope bone scans, and suggested that the pattern of revascularization is of prognostic significance. Revascularization of the epiphysis by a process of recanalization from the lateral margin of the epiphysis had a good prognosis, whereas neovascularization from the base of the epiphysis had a poor prognosis.[70]

PROGNOSTIC FACTORS INFLUENCING THE LONG-TERM OUTCOME

This radiographic classification of Stulberg and colleagues[3] was shown to have clinical relevance; patients with Stulberg Class I and II hips functioned well through adult life, and patients with Class III and IV hips developed symptoms of early degenerative arthritis, forcing some patients to restrict activity during their working life. Patients with Class V hips fared poorly, and most required intervention in the form of an arthroplasty.

Long-term studies have helped to identify the underlying factors in children with Perthes disease that predispose to the development of degenerative arthritis.[3–6] Saito and colleagues[71] demonstrated that steepness of the acetabular roof had a strong association with the onset of degenerative arthritis. However, among various factors that have been implicated, the shape of the femoral head at the time when the disease heals is the most important determinant of the risk for degenerative arthritis.[3–6,71] If the femoral head is spherical when the disease heals it is likely that degenerative arthritis will not develop while if the head is frankly irregular in shape, arthritis will almost certainly ensue. Thus all prognostic factors that determine the shape of the femoral head at healing indirectly influence the long-term outcome.

EVALUATION OF PROGNOSTIC INDICATORS

From the foregoing review the following facts emerge:

- The older the child, the greater the predisposition for femoral head deformation
- The more extensive the epiphyseal infarction, the greater the predisposition for femoral head collapse and deformation
- The greater the epiphyseal collapse (especially the lateral pillar), the greater the predisposition for femoral head deformation
- The presence of abnormalities of the femoral metaphysis and the acetabulum (eg, metaphyseal osteoporosis, metaphyseal cysts, acetabular bicompartmentalization, and so forth) may signal femoral head deformation
- The greater the extrusion of the femoral epiphysis, the greater the predisposition for femoral head deformation.

Of these factors that predispose to femoral head deformation:

- The age of the child is predetermined
- The extent of epiphyseal infarction is predetermined
- The extent of epiphyseal collapse may be prevented but once it occurs, the collapse per se cannot be reversed
- The presence of metaphyseal or acetabular abnormalities cannot be altered by treatment
- Epiphyseal extrusion can be prevented and can be corrected if it develops.

Of the factors that may predispose to femoral head deformation, femoral head extrusion is the most important, and this is the only factor that may be influenced by treatment.

Finally, the relative merits and limitations of prognostic factors discussed in this article are outlined in **Table 2**.

It must be emphasized that any prognostic factor that has been shown to have a strong prognostic significance may be used in retrospective studies to determine factors that may have influenced the outcome of the disease irrespective of when during the disease this factor becomes evident, provided it can be reliably and

Table 2
Evaluation of prognostic factors in Perthes disease

Prognostic Factor	How Reliably Can This Factor be Identified? How Reproducible is it? How Strong is its Prognostic Significance?	When During the Course of the Disease does this Prognostic Factor Become Evident?	Can This Prognostic Factor be Prevented/Reversed/Minimized by Treatment?
Age at onset of the disease	Excellent reproducibility Strong prognostic significance	As soon as disease is diagnosed	No
Gender	Perfect reproducibility Doubtful prognostic significance	As soon as disease is diagnosed	No
Extent of epiphyseal involvement			
Salter-Thompson classification	Good reproducibility (BUT only applicable in one-third of children) Strong prognostic significance	In stage of avascular necrosis (Stage I) if the subchondral fracture line is present	No
Catterall classification	Moderate reproducibility Strong prognostic significance	In the stage of fragmentation (Stage II)	No
Extent of epiphyseal collapse			
Herring classification	Good reproducibility Strong prognostic significance	In the stage of fragmentation (Stage II)	No
Metaphyseal abnormalities			
Metaphyseal cyst	Moderate prognostic significance	In the stage of fragmentation (Stage II)	No
Diffuse metaphyseal reaction	Reproducibility not well tested	In the stage of fragmentation (Stage II)	
Acetabular abnormalities	Moderate prognostic significance Reproducibility not well tested	In the stage of fragmentation (Stage II)	No
Femoral epiphyseal extrusion	Can be reliably and reproducibly identified Strong prognostic significance	Usually commences in the stage of avascular necrosis (Stage I) Frequently clearly identifiable by the early part of the stage of fragmentation (Stage IIa)	Yes It can be prevented by containment before onset of extrusion It can be remedied by containment once extrusion has occurred

reproducibly recognized. However, if a prognostic factor is to be used as a guide to treatment aimed at preventing a poor outcome, it is imperative that it is identified *before* irreversible deformation of the femoral head occurs. See the article by Joseph and Price elsewhere in this issue, it is suggested that deformation of the femoral head often develops by the late stage of fragmentation. Thus if treatment is to be instituted prior to this stage of the disease, several of the prognostic factors cannot be used for decision making even if they have a strong prognostic value simply because they may only be identified later on. In short, the only two prognostic factors that may be identified early enough to institute preventive intervention are femoral head extrusion and the age at onset of the disease.

REFERENCES

1. Catterall A. Legg-Calvé-Perthes disease. Instr Course Lect 1989;38:297–303.
2. Ratliff AH. Perthes' disease. A study of thirty-four hips observed for thirty years. J Bone Joint Surg Br 1967;49(1):102–7.
3. Stulberg SD, Cooperman DR, Wallensten R. The natural history of Legg-Calvé-Perthes disease. J Bone Joint Surg Am 1981;63(7):1095–108.
4. Ippolito E, Tudisco C, Farsetti P. The long-term prognosis of unilateral Perthes' disease. J Bone Joint Surg Br 1987;69(2):243–50.
5. McAndrew MP, Weinstein SL. A long-term follow-up of Legg-Calvé-Perthes disease. J Bone Joint Surg Am 1984;66(6):860–9.
6. Mose K, Hjorth L, Ulfeldt M, et al. Legg Calvé Perthes disease. The late occurrence of coxarthrosis. Acta Orthop Scand Suppl 1977;169:1–39.
7. Mose K. Methods of measuring in Legg-Calvé-Perthes disease with special regard to the prognosis. Clin Orthop Relat Res 1980;150:103–9.
8. Herring JA, Kim HT, Browne R. Legg-Calvé-Perthes disease. Part I: classification of radiographs with use of the modified lateral pillar and Stulberg classifications. J Bone Joint Surg Am 2004;86(10):2103–20.
9. Edgren W. Coxa plana. Acta Orthop Scand Suppl 1965;(Suppl 84):1–129.
10. Harry JD, Gross RH. A quantitative method for evaluating results of treating Legg-Perthes syndrome. J Pediatr Orthop 1987;7(6):671–6.
11. Wiberg G. Studies on dysplastic acetabula and congenital subluxation of the hip joint. With special reference to the complication of osteoarthritis. Acta Chir Scand Suppl 1939;58:7–38.
12. Reimers J. Incidence of full containment of the femoral head after Legg-Calvé-Perthes disease and in the "normal" hip. J Pediatr Orthop 1985; 5(2):199–201.
13. Neyt JG, Weinstein SL, Spratt KF, et al. Stulberg classification system for evaluation of Legg-Calvé-Perthes disease: intra-rater and inter-rater reliability. J Bone Joint Surg Am 1999;81(9): 1209–16.
14. Shah H, Siddesh ND, Joseph B. To what extent does remodeling of the proximal femur and the acetabulum occur between disease healing and skeletal maturity in Perthes disease? A radiological study. J Pediatr Orthop 2008;28(7):711–6.
15. Wiig O, Terjesen T, Svenningsen S. Prognostic factors and outcome of treatment in Perthes' disease: a prospective study of 368 patients with five-year follow-up. J Bone Joint Surg Br 2008; 90(10):1364–71.
16. Nelson D, Zenios M, Ward K, et al. The deformity index as a predictor of final radiological outcome in Perthes' disease. J Bone Joint Surg Br 2007; 89(10):1369–74.
17. Schiller MG, Axer A. Legg-Calvé-Perthes syndrome. A critical analysis of roentgenographic measurements. Clin Orthop 1972;86:34–42.
18. Shah H, Siddesh ND, Joseph B, et al. Effect of prophylactic trochanteric epiphyseodesis in older children with Perthes' disease. J Pediatr Orthop 2009;29(8):889–95.
19. Harris WH. Traumatic arthritis of the hip after dislocation and acetabular fractures: treatment by mold arthroplasty. An end-result study using a new method of result evaluation. J Bone Joint Surg Am 1969;51:737–55.
20. Larson CB. Rating scale for hip disabilities. Clin Orthop Relat Res 1963;31:85–93.
21. Dickens DR, Menelaus MB. The assessment of prognosis in Perthes' disease. J Bone Joint Surg Br 1978;60(2):189–94.
22. Kamegaya M, Saisu T, Miura Y, et al. A proposed prognostic formula for Perthes' disease. Clin Orthop Relat Res 2005;440:205–8.
23. Griffin PP, Green NE, Beauchamp RD. Legg-Calvé-Perthes disease: treatment and prognosis. Orthop Clin North Am 1980;11(1):127–39.
24. Canavese F, Dimeglio A. Perthes' disease: prognosis in children under six years of age. J Bone Joint Surg Br 2008;90(7):940–5.
25. Fabry K, Fabry G, Moens P. Legg-Calvé-Perthes disease in patients under 5 years of age does not always result in a good outcome. Personal experience and meta-analysis of the literature. J Pediatr Orthop B 2003;12(3):222–7.
26. Rosenfeld SB, Herring JA, Chao JC. Legg-Calvé-Perthes disease: a review of cases with onset before six years of age. J Bone Joint Surg Am 2007;89(12): 2712–22.
27. Snyder CR. Legg-Perthes disease in the young hip—does it necessarily do well? J Bone Joint Surg Am 1975;57(6):751–9.

28. Joseph B, Mulpuri K, Varghese G. Perthes' disease in the adolescent. J Bone Joint Surg Br 2001;83(5): 715–20.

29. Specchiulli F, Cofano RE. Long-term follow-up of Perthes' disease in adolescence. Chir Organi Mov 2001;86(1):7–13.

30. Ippolito E, Tudisco C, Farsetti P. Long-term prognosis of Legg-Calvé-Perthes disease developing during adolescence. J Pediatr Orthop 1985;5(6):652–6.

31. Mazda K, Pennecot GF, Zeller R, et al. Perthes' disease after the age of twelve years. Role of the remaining growth. J Bone Joint Surg Br 1999;81(4): 696–8.

32. Evans DL. Legg-Calvé-Perthes' disease. A study of late results. J Bone Joint Surg Br 1958,40.108 81.

33. Guille JT, Lipton GE, Skoze G, et al. Legg-Calvé-Perthes' disease in girls. A comparison of the results with those seen in boys. J Bone Joint Surg Am 1998; 80:1256–63.

34. Catterall A. The natural history of Perthes' disease. J Bone Joint Surg Br 1971;53:37–53.

35. Kamhi E, MacEwen GD. Treatment of Legg-Calvé-Perthes disease. Prognostic value of Catterall's classification. J Bone Joint Surg Am 1975;57(5):651–4.

36. Van Dam BE, Crider RJ, Noyes JD, et al. Determination of the Catterall classification in Legg-Calvé-Perthes disease. J Bone Joint Surg Am 1981;63(6): 906–14.

37. Kamhi E. Legg-Calvé-Perthes disease. Postgrad Med 1976;60(4):125–30.

38. Hardcastle PH, Ross R, Hamalainen M, et al. Catterall grouping of Perthes' disease. An assessment of observer error and prognosis using the Catterall classification. J Bone Joint Surg Br 1980;62:428–31.

39. Christensen F, Soballe K, Ejsted R, et al. The Catterall classification of Perthes' disease: an assessment of reliability. J Bone Joint Surg Br 1986;68(4):614–5.

40. Salter RB, Thompson GH. Legg-Calvé-Perthes disease. The prognostic significance of the subchondral fracture and a two-group classification of the femoral head involvement. J Bone Joint Surg Am 1984;66(4):479–89.

41. Simmons ED, Graham HK, Szalai JP. Interobserver variability in grading Perthes' disease. J Bone Joint Surg Br 1990;72(2):202–4.

42. Mukherjee A, Fabry G. Evaluation of the prognostic indices in Legg-Calvé-Perthes disease: statistical analysis of 116 hips. J Pediatr Orthop 1990;10(2): 153–8.

43. Eyre-Brook AL. Osteochondritis deformans coxae juvenalis or Perthes' disease: the results of treatment by traction in recumbency. Br J Surg 1936;24:166–82.

44. Sjovall H. Zur Frage der Behandlung der Coxa plana. Acta Orthop Scand 1942;13:324–53 [in German].

45. Heyman CH, Herndon CH. Legg-Perthes' disease. A method for measurement of the roentgenographic results. J Bone Joint Surg Am 1950;32:767–78.

46. Heikkinen E, Puranen J. Evaluation of femoral osteotomy in the treatment of Legg-Calvé-Perthes disease. Clin Orthop 1980;150:60–8.

47. Lack W, Feldner-Busztin H, Ritschl P, et al. The results of surgical treatment for Perthes' disease. J Pediatr Orthop 1989;9:197–204.

48. Herring JA, Neustadt JB, Williams JJ, et al. The lateral pillar classification of Legg-Calvé-Perthes disease. J Pediatr Orthop 1992;12:143–50.

49. Ismail AM, Macnicol MF. Prognosis in Perthes' disease: a comparison of radiological predictors. J Bone Joint Surg Br 1998;80(2):310–4.

50. Aksoy MC, Caglar O, Yazici M, et al. Comparison between braced and non-braced Legg-Calvé-Perthes-disease patients: a radiological outcome study. J Pediatr Orthop B 2004;13(3):153 7.

51. Farsetti P, Tudisco C, Caterini R, et al. The Herring lateral pillar classification for prognosis in Perthes disease. Late results in 49 patients treated conservatively. J Bone Joint Surg Br 1995;77(5): 739–42.

52. Gigante C, Frizziero P, Turra S. Prognostic value of Catterall and Herring classification in Legg-Calvé-Perthes disease: follow-up to skeletal maturity of 32 patients. J Pediatr Orthop 2002;22(3): 345–9.

53. Herring JA, Kim HT, Browne R. Legg-Calvé-Perthes disease: part II: prospective multicenter study of the effect of treatment on outcome. J Bone Joint Surg Am 2004;86:2121–34.

54. Lappin K, Kealey D, Cosgrove A. Herring classification: how useful is the initial radiograph? J Pediatr Orthop 2002;22(4):479–82.

55. Langenskiold A. Changes in the capital growth plate and the proximal femoral metaphysis in Legg-Calvé-Perthes disease. Clin Orthop Relat Res 1980;150: 110–4.

56. Robichon J, Desjardins JP, Koch M, et al. The femoral neck in Legg-Perthes' disease. Its relationship to epiphyseal change and its importance in early prognosis. J Bone Joint Surg Br 1974;56(1):62–8.

57. Smith SR, Ions GK, Gregg PJ. The radiological features of the metaphysis in Perthes disease. J Pediatr Orthop 1982;2(4):401–4.

58. Joseph B, Varghese G, Mulpuri K, et al. Natural evolution of Perthes disease: a study of 610 children under 12 years of age at disease onset. J Pediatr Orthop 2003;23(5):590–600.

59. Joseph B. Morphological changes in the acetabulum in Perthes' disease. J Bone Joint Surg Br 1989;71(5):756–63.

60. Danielsson L, Pettersson H, Sunden G. Early assessment of prognosis in Perthes' disease. Acta Orthop Scand 1982;53(4):605–11.

61. Loder RT, Farley FA, Hensinger RN. Physeal slope in Perthes disease. J Bone Joint Surg Br 1995;77(5): 736–8.

62. Murphy RP, Marsh HO. Incidence and natural history of "Head at risk" factors in Perthes' disease. Clin Orthop Relat Res 1978;132:102–7.

63. Gershuni DH. Preliminary evaluation and prognosis in Legg-Calvé-Perthes disease. Clin Orthop Relat Res 1980;150.16–22.

64. Joseph B, Rao N, Mulpuri K, et al. How does a femoral varus osteotomy alter the natural evolution of Perthes' disease? J Pediatr Orthop 2005;14(1):10–5.

65. Green NE, Beauchamp RD, Griffin PP. Epiphyseal extrusion as a prognostic index in Legg-Calvé-Perthes disease. J Bone Joint Surg Am 1981;63(6):900–5.

66. de Sanctis N, Rega AN, Rondinella F. Prognostic evaluation of Legg-Calvé-Perthes disease by MRI. Part I: the role of physeal involvement. J Pediatr Orthop 2000;20(4):455–62.

67. de Sanctis N, Rondinella F. Prognostic evaluation of Legg-Calvé-Perthes disease by MRI. Part II: pathomorphogenesis and new classification. J Pediatr Orthop 2000;20(4):463–70.

68. Shigeno Y, Evans GA. Revised arthrographic index of deformity for Perthes' disease. J Pediatr Orthop B 1996;5(1):44–7.

69. Shigeno Y, Evans GA. Quantitative correlation between the initial and final femoral head deformity in Perthes' disease. J Pediatr Orthop B 1996;5(1):48–54.

70. Conway JJ. A scintigraphic classification of Legg-Calvé-Perthes disease. Semin Nucl Med 1993;23(4):274–95.

71. Saito S, Takaoka K, Ono K, et al. Residual deformities related to arthrotic change after Perthes' disease. A long-term follow-up of fifty-one cases. Arch Orthop Trauma Surg 1985;104(1):7–14.

Principles of Containment Treatment Aimed at Preventing Femoral Head Deformation in Perthes Disease

Benjamin Joseph, MS Orth, MCh Orth[a],*,
Charles T. Price, MD[b,c]

KEYWORDS

• Perthes disease • Containment • Femoral head deformation
• Prevention

WHY TREAT PERTHES?

Perthes disease is a self-limiting disease in children; the interruption of the blood supply to the femoral epiphysis is temporary and complete revascularization of the epiphysis is the norm if the child is younger than 12 years at onset of the disease.[1,2] No treatment is needed to facilitate the process of revascularization. As the blood supply to the epiphysis is reestablished, the necrotic bone is completely replaced by healthy new bone by a process of "creeping substitution" (**Fig. 1**).[3,4] This raises the question "why do we need to treat children with Perthes disease?"

Treatment is needed in some children in whom the femoral head may become deformed while revascularization proceeds over a period of 2 to 4 years. Treatment of these susceptible children should ideally be directed to attempting to prevent the femoral head from becoming deformed.

To plan an appropriate strategy for preventive treatment it is imperative that one understands what causes the femoral head to become deformed and when during the evolution of the disease irreversible deformation of the femoral head occurs.

HOW DOES FEMORAL HEAD DEFORMATION OCCUR?

Following the vascular insult part or all of the femoral epiphysis becomes necrotic; this triggers a synovitis,[5–7] articular cartilage hypertrophy,[8] and hypertrophy of the ligamentum teres.[9] These soft tissue changes compounded by muscle spasm cause the femoral head to extrude beyond the acetabular margin. Weight-bearing stresses and forces of muscular contraction are transmitted across the acetabular margin onto the extruded part of the femoral head. While normal healthy bone can quite effectively withstand these physiologic stresses, bone of the avascular epiphysis is not capable of withstanding them.[10,11] If more than 20% of the width of the epiphysis extrudes outside the acetabular margin, there is a very high risk of irreversible femoral head deformation (**Fig. 2**).[12,13]

The author has nothing to disclose.
[a] Department of Orthopaedics, Kasturba Medical College, Manipal 576 104, Karnataka State, India
[b] Pediatric Orthopaedic Division, Arnold Palmer Hospital for Children, 83 West Columbia Street, Orlando, FL 32806, USA
[c] Orthopedic Surgery, University of Central Florida College of Medicine, 6850 Lake Nona Boulevard, Orlando, FL 32827, USA
* Corresponding author.
E-mail address: bjosephortho@yahoo.co.in

Orthop Clin N Am 42 (2011) 317–327
doi:10.1016/j.ocl.2011.04.001
0030-5898/11/$ – see front matter © 2011 Elsevier Inc. All rights reserved.

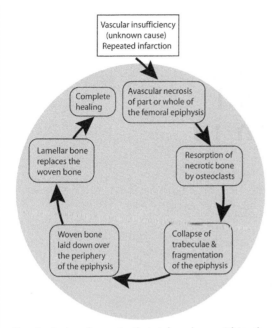

Fig. 1. Cycle of events that take place within the femoral epiphysis in Perthes disease.

Extrusion appears to be the most important factor that predisposes to femoral head deformation.

WHEN DOES FEMORAL HEAD DEFORMATION OCCUR?

The disease was first divided by Waldenstrom[14] into two stages, based on plain radiographic appearance: an initial evolutionary stage and a later stage of healing. Subsequently investigators divided the disease into 4 stages: the stage of avascular necrosis, the stage of fragmentation, the stage of reconstitution or regeneration, and the healed stage. More recently the first 3 stages were further divided into early and late stages (**Fig. 3**),[13] thus enabling clinicians to define the timing of events leading to femoral head deformation more clearly.

It was noted that in untreated children femoral head extrusion increased modestly through the initial stages of the disease, but abruptly increased as they reached the late stage of fragmentation, often exceeding 20% (**Fig. 4**).[13] This finding clearly suggests that the predilection for deformation increases once the disease evolves to this stage.

The epiphysis is most vulnerable to deformation during the late stage of fragmentation and in the early part of the stage of reconstitution. The reason for the vulnerability varies in these two stages. In the late stage of fragmentation the necrotic bone is being actively resorbed and the dead trabeculae are thus weakened and prone to collapse. On the other hand, in the early stage of reconstitution viable trabeculae of the woven bone that is newly laid down on the periphery of the epiphysis are also prone to collapse, because the bony trabeculae are initially laid down haphazardly and not in the direction that enables them to resist stress. Until the woven bone is replaced by mature lamellar bone (with trabeculae aligned so as to resist compressive and tensile forces), this propensity for deformation will persist (**Fig. 5**).

The impression that femoral head deformation occurs either at the late stage of fragmentation or soon thereafter is supported by the observation that the metaphysis widens quite abruptly at this stage.[13] Marked widening of the metaphysis suggests that the femoral head is flattened and that coxa magna is going to develop, as there is a strong correlation between metaphyseal width during the course of Perthes disease and the size of the femoral head at skeletal maturity.

THE TIMELINE OF TREATMENT OF PERTHES DISEASE

Because it is clear that femoral head deformation tends to occur around the late stage of fragmentation, this stage divides the cycle of evolution of the disease into two distinct parts; the stages

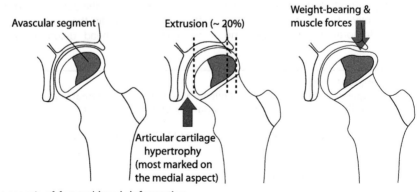

Fig. 2. Pathogenesis of femoral head deformation.

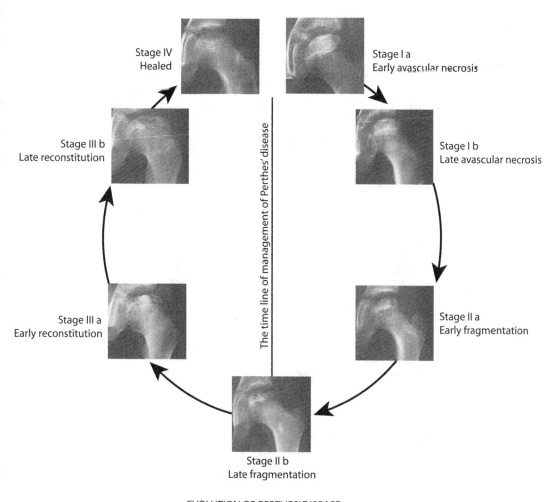

Stage IV
Healed

Stage I a
Early avascular necrosis

Stage III b
Late reconstitution

Stage I b
Late avascular necrosis

The time line of management of Perthes' disease

Stage III a
Early reconstitution

Stage II a
Early fragmentation

Stage II b
Late fragmentation

EVOLUTION OF PERTHES' DISEASE

Fig. 3. Stages of evolution of Perthes disease and the time line of management.

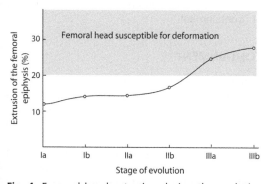

Fig. 4. Femoral head extrusion during the evolution of the disease. (*Data from* Joseph B, Varghese G, Mulpuri K, et al. Natural evolution of Perthes disease: a study of 610 children under 12 years of age at disease onset. J Pediatr Orthop 2003;23(5):590–600.)

preceding this point form the early part of the disease cycle (see **Fig. 3**).

More importantly, this line defines when treatment aimed at preventing femoral head deformation is likely to succeed. Any preventive intervention is justified only from the onset of the disease to the early stage of fragmentation. Treatment instituted at the late stage of fragmentation or thereafter is either remedial in nature or frankly salvage in nature (**Fig. 6**).

THE AIM OF TREATMENT OF PERTHES EARLY IN THE COURSE OF THE DISEASE

The aim of treatment of Perthes in the early part of the disease is to prevent the femoral head from becoming deformed by muscular forces and weight-bearing stresses transmitted across the acetabular margin.

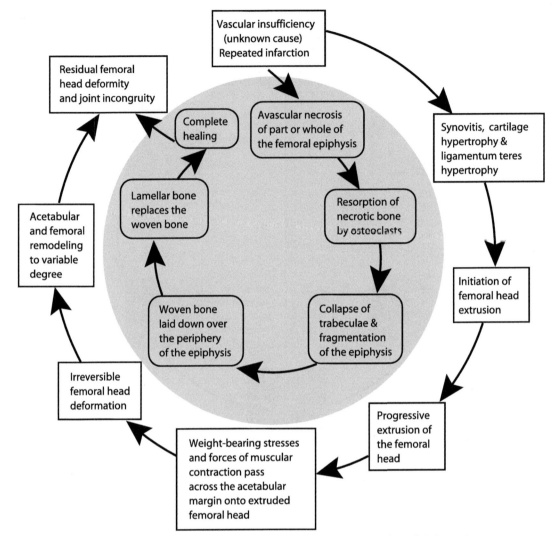

Fig. 5. Cycles of events that determine the timing and predilection to femoral head deformation.

WHAT ARE THE TREATMENT OPTIONS?

There are 3 theoretical options for treatment directed toward preventing femoral head deformation.

1. The first approach attempts to prevent the femoral head from bearing forces across the acetabular margin by either preventing or reversing extrusion of the femoral head.
2. The second attempts to minimize stress on the femoral head by avoiding bearing weight on the limb.
3. The third, relatively novel approach, which is still experimental, attempts to prevent the bone from becoming weak by reducing the osteoclastic resorption of the necrotic bone (see article by Little and Kim elsewhere in this issue).

The first of these options is what is most widely practiced currently, and is based on the principle of "containment."

CONTAINMENT

Containment is the term used to describe intervention that ensures that the anterolateral part of the femoral epiphysis is positioned within the acetabulum, thereby protecting the epiphysis from being subjected to deforming stresses.

Containment can be achieved by two different methods. The first involves positioning the femur either in abduction and internal rotation or in abduction and flexion (**Fig. 7**), which can be done by casting, bracing, or surgery on the femur. Alternatively, containment can be achieved by an osteotomy of the pelvis that reorients the

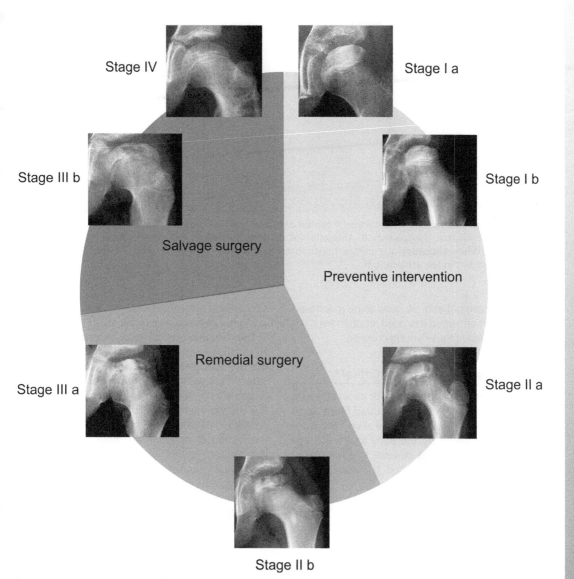

Stage IV

Stage I a

Stage III b

Stage I b

Salvage surgery

Preventive intervention

Remedial surgery

Stage III a

Stage II a

Stage II b

Fig. 6. Treatment options in different stages of evolution of Perthes disease.

acetabulum such that it covers the anterolateral part of the femoral epiphysis (eg, Salter osteotomy, triple innominate osteotomy) or by creating a bony shelf over the extruded part of the epiphysis.

Who Needs Containment?

Because containment is treatment aimed at correcting or preventing femoral head extrusion, the decision to offer containment should be governed by the propensity for femoral head extrusion in the child in question.

In children older than 8 years at the onset of the disease, extrusion invariably occurs sooner or later in the course of the disease,[13,15] hence containment should be offered as soon as the disease is diagnosed.

In children younger than 8 years at the onset of the disease, the likelihood of extrusion development is uncertain; these children need to be monitored closely and containment offered as soon as extrusion is detected. Once extrusion is detected, delaying intervention is not justifiable because extrusion increases as the disease evolves (see **Fig. 4**; **Fig. 8**).

Although a major proportion of children who are younger than 5 years at the onset of the disease has a favorable prognosis, it must not be assumed that all children younger than 5 years will necessarily

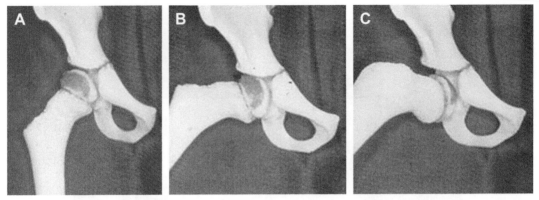

Fig. 7. Model to illustrate how containment can be obtained. (*A*) The area marked red depicts the part of the avascular epiphysis that is extruded. (*B*) Abduction of the hip facilitates containment of the lateral part of the epiphysis. (*C*) When abduction is combined with internal rotation, the anterior part of the epiphysis is also well contained within the acetabulum.

do well.[16] These patients do need to be monitored and, if the femoral head extrudes, containment will be needed even in these young children.

Is the Timing of Containment Critical?

If containment treatment is to work as an effective method of preventing the femoral head from becoming deformed, it is imperative that containment is achieved by the early stage of fragmentation (ie, before the disease evolves to the point where the femoral head is vulnerable for deformation; **Fig. 9**).

This contention is supported by the observation that the extent of epiphyseal extrusion at the late stage of fragmentation has a very strong association with the shape of the femoral head when the disease heals (**Fig. 10**).[13]

The importance of early containment was emphasized repeatedly by several investigators, but this has often not been heeded. Axer advocated containment "in the early stage of the disease."[17,18] Heikkinen and Puranen[19] suggested that containment "should be done as early as possible." Hiokka and colleagues[20] noted that the results of containment were poor if done in the healing phase of the disease. Lack and colleagues[21] observed that containment "in the condensation stage" was far more effective than containment later in the course of the disease. Although each of these investigators used different terms to describe the early stages of the disease,

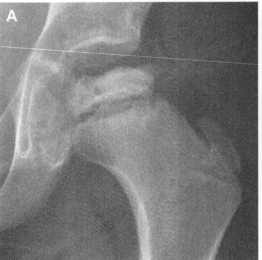
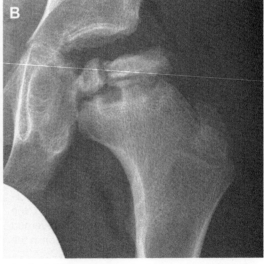

Fig. 8. (*A*) Early extrusion of the femoral head is evident in the left hip of a 7-year-old boy. Containment was deferred. (*B*) Four months later, extrusion has clearly become worse.

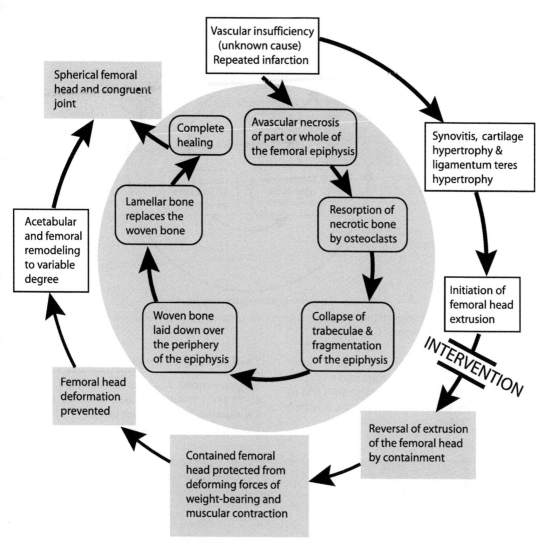

Fig. 9. The effects of appropriate timing of intervention to prevent the femoral head from getting deformed.

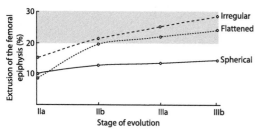

Fig. 10. The effect of extrusion of the femoral head on the shape of the femoral head at healing in untreated cases of Perthes disease. If extrusion is not corrected by stage IIb the femoral head is likely to deform. Mean values are shown; the shaded area indicates extrusion in excess of 20%. (*Data from* Joseph B, Varghese G, Mulpuri K, et al. Natural evolution of Perthes disease: a study of 610 children under 12 years of age at disease onset. J Pediatr Orthop 2003;23(5): 590–600.)

the message was the same. The recommendations for early intervention in some of these earlier reports were not based on robust statistical analysis, but they are now supported by a study showing that the odds ratio of avoiding femoral head deformation is 16.58 times higher if containment is achieved early in the disease (stage IIa or earlier) than if it is achieved late in the disease (stage IIb or later).[22]

Prerequisites for Containment

It is imperative that an adequate range of motion is present when containment treatment is instituted, as satisfactory containment cannot be achieved if the hip is stiff. A short period of traction often relieves muscle spasm in children with restricted motion. Another method of restoring motion is to apply abduction casts and increase the abduction

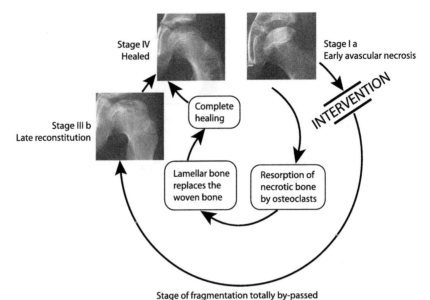

Fig. 11. Altered natural history of the disease in children who undergo varus osteotomy in the stage of avascular necrosis and bypass the stage of fragmentation.

every 2 weeks until a satisfactory range of motion is obtained. In the more recalcitrant hips an abduction cast applied under general anesthesia and retained for 6 weeks usually resolves the irritability and restores motion.

The End Point of Containment

Surgical means achieves containment, and the effect lasts throughout the vulnerable period of the disease. However, the containment effect of bracing or casting is present only as long as the

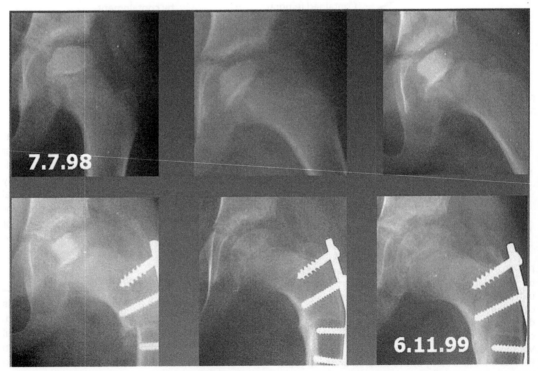

Fig. 12. Serial radiographs of an 8-year-old boy who had a varus osteotomy performed in the stage of avascular necrosis. The stage of fragmentation was bypassed, and the disease healed in 16 months.

device is worn, which raises the question: how long should casting or bracing be continued? In the foregoing sections of this article it has been emphasized that femoral head deformation occurs in either the late stage of fragmentation (stage IIb) or the early stage of reconstitution (stage IIIa). It follows that containment should be maintained until the disease has progressed beyond this point (ie, bracing or casting should continue until the onset of stage IIIb) but need not be continued until complete healing of the disease has occurred.[23]

What are the Effects of Containment?

The results of various forms of containment treatment reported in the literature suggest that it does improve the chances of retaining the sphericity of the femoral head in children with Perthes disease.[24–28] In addition, the extent of femoral head enlargement and the severity of coxa magna can be reduced by containment.[28]

Because surgical containment involves an osteotomy of the femur or pelvis, it is possible that this may have an effect on the healing process itself. It was generally assumed that these forms of bony surgery did not influence the rate of healing of the disease.[29,30] However, when a femoral varus osteotomy is performed during the stage of avascular necrosis, the stage of fragmentation is bypassed in one-third of the operated children (**Fig. 11**).[28,31] The duration of the disease is clearly reduced in these children, and what is most gratifying is that every one of these children had spherical hips when the disease had healed (**Fig. 12**).

Weight Relief

There is very little evidence in the literature to support weight relief in isolation as a method of

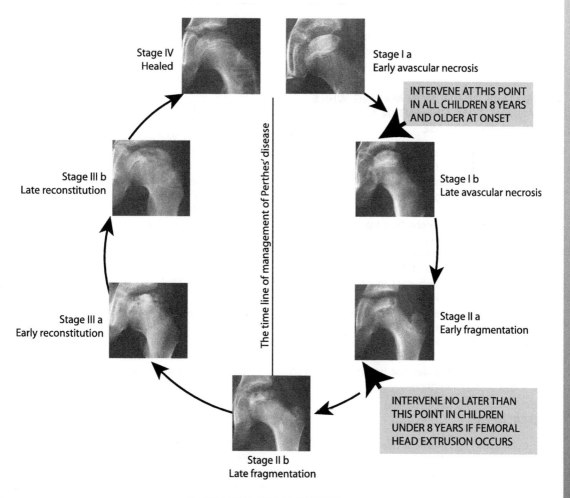

Stage IV
Healed

Stage I a
Early avascular necrosis

INTERVENE AT THIS POINT IN ALL CHILDREN 8 YEARS AND OLDER AT ONSET

Stage III b
Late reconstitution

Stage I b
Late avascular necrosis

The time line of management of Perthes' disease

Stage III a
Early reconstitution

Stage II a
Early fragmentation

INTERVENE NO LATER THAN THIS POINT IN CHILDREN UNDER 8 YEARS IF FEMORAL HEAD EXTRUSION OCCURS

Stage II b
Late fragmentation

EVOLUTION OF PERTHES' DISEASE

Fig. 13. Optimal timing of containment in children with Perthes disease determined by the age at onset of symptoms.

Table 1
Outline of decision making for instituting containment treatment early in the course of Perthes disease (ie, in stages Ia, Ib, or IIa)

Factors to Consider Early in the Course of Perthes Disease			
Age at Onset	Extrusion of Femoral Head	Range of Motion	Recommended Treatment
Under 8 years	Absent	Good	• No containment • Preserve range of motion • Monitor for extrusion with radiographs every 4 months
	Present	Good Poor	• Contain as soon as possible • Restore motion by traction/abduction cast for 6 weeks • Treat by containment once motion is restored
8 years and older	Present or absent (ie, irrespective of whether extrusion is present or not)	Good Poor	• Contain as soon as possible • Restore motion by traction/abduction cast for 6 weeks • Treat by containment once motion is restored

treatment for Perthes disease. However, some reports suggest that combining weight relief with containment may be beneficial.[32]

SUMMARY OF DECISION MAKING WHILE PLANNING CONTAINMENT IN THE EARLY PART OF THE DISEASE

The factors to take into consideration when deciding on treatment include the age of the child at the onset of symptoms (**Fig. 13**), the presence of extrusion of the femoral head, and the range of motion of the hip.

The outline of treatment that takes these variables into consideration is shown in **Table 1**.

The two factors that have been used widely for decision making (ie, the status of the lateral pillar and the extent of epiphyseal involvement) have not been included in the decision-making scheme, as often treatment may need to be initiated well before these two variables can be identified with some degree of certainty; this is because Catterall's grouping and Herring's grading can be applied only once the disease has progressed to the stage of fragmentation.

REFERENCES

1. Catterall A. Legg-Calvé-Perthes syndrome. Clin Orthop Relat Res 1981;158:41–52.
2. Conway JJ. A scintigraphic classification of Legg-Calvé-Perthes disease. Semin Nucl Med 1993;23(4):274–95.
3. Jensen OM, Lauritzen J. Legg-Calvé-Perthes' disease. Morphological studies in two cases examined at necropsy. J Bone Joint Surg Br 1976;58(3):332–8.
4. Salter RB. Legg-Calvé-Perthes disease: the scientific basis for the methods of treatment and their indications. Clin Orthop Relat Res 1980;150:8–11.
5. Howarth MB. Coxa plana. J Bone Joint Surg Am 1948;30:601–20.
6. Matsoukas JA. Viral antibody titres to rubella in coxa plana or Perthes' disease. Perthes disease: is it the late osseous residua of minor prenatal rubella? Acta Orthop Scand 1975;46:957–62.
7. Joseph B, Pydisetty RK. Chondrolysis and the stiff hip in Perthes' disease: an immunological study. J Pediatr Orthop 1996;16(1):15–9.
8. Joseph B. Morphological changes in the acetabulum in Perthes' disease. J Bone Joint Surg Br 1989;71(5):756–63.
9. Kamegaya M, Moriya H, Tsuchiya K, et al. Arthrography of early Perthes' disease. Swelling of the ligamentum teres as a cause of subluxation. J Bone Joint Surg Br 1989;71(3):413–7.
10. Rab GT, DeNatale JS, Herrmann LR. Three-dimensional finite element analysis of Legg-Calvé-Perthes disease. J Pediatr Orthop 1982;2(1):39–44.
11. Ueo T, Tsutsumi S, Yamamuro T, et al. Biomechanical analysis of Perthes' disease using the finite element method: the role of swelling of articular cartilage. Arch Orthop Trauma Surg 1987;106(4):202–8.
12. Griffin PP, Green NE, Beauchamp RD. Legg-Calvé-Perthes disease: treatment and prognosis. Orthop Clin North Am 1980;11(1):127–39.
13. Joseph B, Varghese G, Mulpuri K, et al. Natural evolution of Perthes disease: a study of 610 children under 12 years of age at disease onset. J Pediatr Orthop 2003;23(5):590–600.

14. Waldenstrom H. The first stages of coxa plana. J Bone Joint Surg Am 1938;20:559–66.

15. Muirhead-Allwood W, Catterall A. The treatment of Perthes' disease. The results of a trial of management. J Bone Joint Surg Br 1982;64(3):282–5.

16. Fabry K, Fabry G, Moens P. Legg-Calvé-Perthes disease in patients under 5 years of age does not always result in a good outcome. Personal experience and meta-analysis of the literature. J Pediatr Orthop B 2003;12(3):222–7.

17. Axer A. Subtrochanteric osteotomy in the treatment of Perthes' disease: a preliminary report. J Bone Joint Surg Br 1965;47:489–99.

18. Axer A, Gershuni DH, Hendel D, et al. Indications for femoral osteotomy in Legg-Calvé-Perthes disease. Clin Orthop Relat Res 1980;150:78–87.

19. Heikkinen E, Puranen J. Evaluation of femoral osteotomy in the treatment of Legg-Calvé-Perthes disease. Clin Orthop Relat Res 1980;150:60–8.

20. Hoikka V, Poussa M, Yrjonen T, et al. Intertrochanteric varus osteotomy for Perthes' disease. Radiographic changes after 2–16-year follow-up of 126 hips. Acta Orthop Scand 1991;62(6):549–53.

21. Lack W, Feldner-Busztin H, Ritschl P, et al. The results of surgical treatment for Perthes' disease. J Pediatr Orthop 1989;9(2):197–204.

22. Joseph B, Nair NS, Narasimha Rao KL, et al. Optimal timing for containment surgery for Perthes' disease. J Pediatr Orthop 2003;23(5):601–6.

23. Thompson GH, Westin GW. Legg-Calvé-Perthes disease: results of discontinuing treatment in the early reossification phase. Clin Orthop Relat Res 1979;139:70–80.

24. Herring J, Kim MT, Browne R. Legg-Calvé-Perthes disease: part II: prospective multicenter study of the effect of treatment on outcome. J Bone Joint Surg Am 2004;86:2121–34,

25. Stevens PM, Williams P, Menelaus M. Innominate osteotomy for Perthes' disease. J Pediatr Orthop 1981;1(1):47–54.

26. Paterson DC, Leitch JM, Foster BK. Results of innominate osteotomy in the treatment of Legg-Calvé-Perthes disease. Clin Orthop Relat Res 1991;266:96–103.

27. Wiig O, Terjesen T, Svenningsen S. Prognostic factors and outcome of treatment in Perthes' disease. J Bone Joint Surg Br 2008;90:1364–71.

28. Joseph B, Rao N, Mulpuri K, et al. How does a femoral varus osteotomy alter the natural evolution of Perthes' disease? J Pediatr Orthop B 2005;14(1):10–5.

29. Marklund T, Tillberg B. Coxa plana: a radiological comparison of the rate of healing with conservative measures and after osteotomy. J Bone Joint Surg Br 1976;58:25–30.

30. Iwasaki K. The change in venous circulation of the proximal part of the femur after varus osteotomy in Perthes' disease. Nippon Seikeigeka Gakkai Zasshi 1986;60:237–49.

31. Wichlacz W, Sotirow B, Sionek A, et al. The surgical treatment of children with Perthes' disease: 26 years of experience. Ortop Traumatol Rehabil 2004;6(6):718–27.

32. Mintowt-Czyz W, Tayton K. Indication for weight relief and containment in the treatment of Perthes' disease. Acta Orthop Scand 1983;54(3):439–45.

Containment Methods for Treatment of Legg-Calvé-Perthes Disease

Charles T. Price, MD[a,b],*, George H. Thompson, MD[c,d], Dennis R. Wenger, MD[e]

KEYWORDS
- Perthes disease • Containment • Lateral migration
- Osteotomy

The objective of containment treatment in Perthes disease is to hold the femoral head in the acetabulum during the period of "biologic plasticity" while necrotic bone is resorbed and living bone is restored through the process of "creeping substitution."[1] This prevents lateral migration of the femoral head and thereby avoids flattening while the necrotic bone is being replaced with living bone. To be successful, it is best to initiate containment while the femoral head is still round.[2] This is during the period of preventive intervention that was identified in the preceding article on principles of containment treatment elsewhere in this issue. During the late fragmentation stage, containment may not be possible because of hinged abduction. Hinge abduction in the fragmentation stage requires different strategies for treatment other than containment. Also, containment is no longer beneficial after the fragmentation stage, or when the femoral head is already enlarged, partially healed, and permanently deformed.

The dilemma in Perthes disease is that some patients do not require treatment, but outcomes are better when the decision to treat is made early in the course of the disorder. During these early stages it is difficult to classify the severity of involvement by current systems of classification.

AGE AT ONSET

For clarity of definition, two issues should be emphasized. First, it should be noted that it is the age at onset of symptoms that is to be taken into consideration and not the age at presentation to the surgeon. Second, chronologic age has been used in almost all natural history studies and this sometimes causes confusion. A child who has had his eighth birthday is older than 8 years of age and can also be considered younger than 9 years of age. This is similar to the description of a 2-month old infant who would be considered older than zero but younger than 1 year of age. After the first birthday he or she will be older than 1 year but younger than 2 years.

The child's age at onset of symptoms can provide guidance to initial planning in many cases.

[a] Pediatric Orthopaedic Division, Arnold Palmer Hospital for Children, 83 West Columbia Street, Orlando, FL 32806, USA
[b] Orthopedic Surgery, University of Central Florida College of Medicine, 6850 Lake Nona Boulevard, Orlando, FL 32827, USA
[c] Pediatric Orthopaedics, Rainbow Babies & Children's Hospital, 11100 Euclid Avenue, Cleveland, OH 44106, USA
[d] Orthopaedic Surgery and Pediatrics Case Western Reserve University, 2109 Adelbert Road, Cleveland, OH 44106, USA
[e] Department of Orthopaedic Surgery, Rady Children's Hospital San Diego, University of California San Diego, 3030 Children's Way, Suite 410, San Diego, CA 92103, USA
* Corresponding author. Pediatric Orthopaedic Division, Arnold Palmer Hospital for Children, 83 West Columbia Street Orlando, FL 32806.
E-mail address: charles.price@orlandohealth.com

Orthop Clin N Am 42 (2011) 329–340
doi:10.1016/j.ocl.2011.04.008
0030-5898/11/$ – see front matter © 2011 Elsevier Inc. All rights reserved.

Long-term studies indicate that untreated children 9 years and older at onset of symptoms have a poor prognosis regardless of extent of involvement of the capital femoral epiphysis. Also, before lateral pillar collapse, children 8 years and older (or with bone age older than 6 years in boys) have improved outcomes following surgical intervention compared with nonoperative treatments.[3] Children younger than 5 years at onset have a low risk of early osteoarthritis.[4,5] Some children in this age group do develop poor radiographic outcomes, but the prognosis is similar whether these younger children are treated by observation or by surgical containment.[6,7] Growth disturbances rather than femoral head collapse may contribute to some of these poor results in younger children, but growth disturbance may not be influenced by containment. Therefore, children younger than 5 years rarely benefit from treatment other than brief limitation of activities for symptomatic management. Children between 5 and 8 years at onset should be contained early in the course of disease when the extent of femoral head involvement is clearly greater than 50% (Catterall 3–4). Other cases in the 5- to 8-year age group may be observed to determine whether the hip will spontaneously remain contained or whether lateral migration (eccentration) develops.

LATERAL MIGRATION

Lateral migration is associated with poor outcomes.[8] For this reason, the authors recommend containment between the ages of 5 and 8 years as soon as lateral migration is identified. When early lateral migration is identified in this age group, containment is advisable before development of femoral head deformity and hinge abduction. For patients 8 years or older at onset of symptoms, containment is recommended as soon as the diagnosis is confirmed rather than waiting for signs of lateral migration, because the prognosis is poor for children in this age group.[9]

METHODS OF CONTAINMENT

It is our opinion that all forms of containment can be successful when containment is initiated early in the course of disease and the principles of that particular method of containment are followed appropriately. There are advantages and disadvantages of almost all forms of containment. When a method of containment is selected for an individual patient, it is generally best to stay with that method rather than changing later in the course of disease. Some of the current literature includes outcomes of containment methods that were selected after the initial method of containment failed. This article identifies the various methods of containment and the technical aspects of each method. Choice of method depends on the experience of the surgeon and the psychosocial needs of the patient and family. Failure is more commonly a result of inappropriate patient selection for a particular method, delay in management, or technical errors rather than to the method that was selected.

Bed Rest and Range of Motion Treatment

Bed rest and physiotherapy can improve range of motion in most patients.[10] However, this is considered noncontainment treatment and has not improved outcomes.[11,12] Treatment to restore range of motion without containment surgery has been less successful than containment surgery in children 8 years and older.[3] Terjesen and colleagues[13] considered treatment with bed rest and range of motion to represent the natural history of untreated Legg-Calvé-Perthes disease. Decreased hip motion early in the course of disease is generally caused by muscle, owing to the subchondral fracture. In later stages, deformity of the femoral head or true muscle contracture may limit movement.[14] Thus, limitation of motion before femoral head deformity may represent a symptom of severity rather than a cause of pathologic progression.

Pain relief by bed rest may reduce muscle spasm, but does little to prevent deformity of the femoral head. Successful range of motion treatment may indicate milder Perthes disease, especially in younger children. Failed range of motion treatment may indicate more severe Perthes disease with persistent muscle spasm and subsequent femoral head deformity. Thus, physical therapy and bed rest may select only the milder cases whereas moderate to severe patients are subjected to delayed containment treatment. Bed rest and range of motion therapy may help relieve symptoms in preparation for containment treatment, but the authors do not recommend bed rest and physical therapy as a form of definitive treatment for Perthes disease.

Containment by Casts and Bracing

The outcomes of Petrie casts and bracing combined with limited ambulation have been successful when used for prolonged periods.[15–17] Containment can be achieved by nonoperative methods when the braces or casts include the thigh and leg with hip abduction and moderate internal rotation.[18] This must be maintained until the fragmentation stage is complete, all necrotic bone has been resorbed, and there is early sub-chondral bone formation. The time for this to occur is 12 to 18 months from onset of symptoms depending on the age of the child.[19] One advantage of this method is that hospitalization is not required. The major disadvantage is the limited mobility and prolonged treatment time.

Petrie casts or a custom lower extremity A-frame orthotic can hold the lower extremities in wide abduction and slight internal rotation with the knees slightly flexed (**Fig. 1**). These can be removed for bathing, but can also be removed inappropriately by the patient. Limited ambulation may be possible when the knees are included for proper containment, but community mobility requires a wheelchair with removable side arms. Tilting the lower extremities is necessary to enter standard doorways. This lengthy treatment is difficult in a mobile society when both parents may be working outside the home and patients are no longer admitted to pediatric rehabilitation hospitals for treatment of Perthes disease. Another disadvantage is that patients may become non-compliant and then choose surgery in later stages of femoral head collapse when surgical containment may be less successful.

Ambulatory brace treatment for Perthes disease has declined in use for a number of reasons. Primarily, the outcomes of ambulatory bracing have been inferior to surgical containment for patients older than 8 years at onset.[3] Reasons for inferior outcomes may include noncompliance during prolonged brace treatment, braces that fail to control abduction, or concerns about behavioral sequelae (**Fig. 2**).[20,21] The Atlanta Scottish Rite abduction orthosis and weight-relieving abduction braces have largely been abandoned because studies have shown little improvement compared with the natural history of Perthes disease.[21–23]

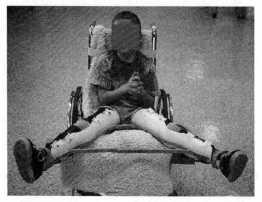

Fig. 1. A child in a lower extremity A-frame orthotic to hold the lower extremities in wide abduction as a method of containment.

Weight-relieving braces that do not contain the hip may promote subluxation and increase pressure on the lateral aspect of the femoral head.[24]

For children younger than 8 years at onset, the outcomes of brace treatment and surgical containment are approximately equal.[3,7] Before the age of 5 years, treatment may not influence outcome.[6,7] For children aged 6 to 8 years, Herring and colleagues[3] reported a slight trend toward improved outcomes of bracing and surgery compared with no treatment, but this difference was not statistically significant. There was no difference in the 6-year to 8-year age group between treatment with braces or surgery.

Restoration of range of motion is necessary before a brace or cast can be expected to contain the hip in Perthes disease. Petrie casts can be applied in the clinic with gradually increasing abduction. It is recommended that casts be removed every 6 to 8 weeks for 24 to 48 hours to restore range of motion to the knees before another cast is applied. Alternatively, traction with bed rest or with slings and springs may be used to restore motion.[25] Oral anti-inflammatory medications may also be helpful, but the role of physical therapy is questionable.[26] After range of motion has been restored, full-time bracing is required except for bathing purposes. This must be continued for 12 to 18 months until all dense, necrotic bone has been resorbed. This indicates the end of the fragmentation stage and beginning of re-ossification. It is safe to discontinue bracing at this stage even though the femoral head is not fully re-ossified.[19]

In summary, it is the authors' opinion that cast and brace treatment may improve outcomes in the age group of 5 to 8 years at time of onset. The method should include restoration of motion followed by immobilization of the leg, knee, and thigh in abduction with limited weight bearing. This should be continued for approximately 12 to 18 months. It is not recommended to attempt this form of containment with the intention of performing surgery if braces or casts fail. That would delay definitive containment until later stages when any method of containment would be less effective.

Containment by Proximal Femoral Varus Osteotomy

There have been numerous reports of containment by proximal femoral varus osteotomy since Axer reported this method in 1965.[27] When compared with the Salter and other rotational pelvic osteotomies, the outcomes are approximately equal.[3,28] Both procedures should be performed in the early stages of disease but the rotational pelvic osteotomies require a spherical femoral head and full

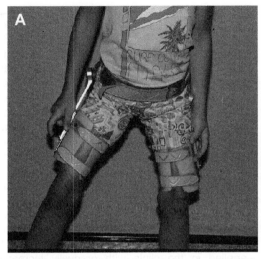
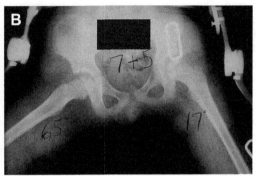

Fig. 2. (*A*) A child in Atlanta hip abduction brace. (*B*) The radiograph in the brace shows that this orthosis fails to abduct the affected hip.

range of motion preoperatively. The proximal femoral varus osteotomy may be less suitable for children 9 years and older because remodeling is unreliable.[25,29,30]

Proximal femoral varus osteotomy can be performed when range of motion is moderately restricted because it shortens the femur, reduces joint reaction forces, and medializes the direction of those forces.[31] Another advantage of femoral varus osteotomy is that it is a familiar procedure for most pediatric orthopedic surgeons. Abnormal venous congestion in the proximal femur is relieved by proximal femoral osteotomy, but the effect on rate of healing of the femoral head may be variable.[32–34] Joseph and colleagues[34] noted acceleration of healing when proximal femoral varus osteotomy was performed early in the course of disease.

The major disadvantage of proximal femoral varus osteotomy is the potential for residual shortening with coxa brevis and trochanteric prominence. This is more likely to occur when the patient is 8 years or older.[25,28,35] Abductor limp and femoral shortening in the early postoperative period may cause concern for parents. However, these resolve in most patients because of remodeling and growth stimulation (**Fig. 3**).[35–37] Growth disturbance of the femoral neck in Perthes disease is the most likely cause of persistent coxa brevis instead of inadequate remodeling in children younger than 8 years.[38] When a Salter osteotomy or shelf procedure is performed, shortening and trochanteric prominence are uncommon. This may be because proximal femoral varus osteotomy creates varus and shortening that are more problematic when growth disturbances

develop.[28,37,38] Attention to technical details and appropriate selection of patients can minimize the risks of shortening and coxa vara.

The authors consider proximal femoral varus osteotomy a useful form of containment for children who meet the criteria for containment, as previously noted. The major technical considerations are to restore at least 30° of abduction in extension before surgery,[25,26,39] and to preserve a neck-shaft angle of 110° with the desired neck-shaft angle being approximately 115°.[26,40,41]

Additional technical considerations include the following:

1. Perform no more than 20° of varus. Kim and colleagues[41] noted that 15° of varus is sufficient.
2. Perform opening wedge osteotomy to reduce limb length discrepancy.[35]
3. Add approximately 15° of extension to the osteotomy to help contain the anterior aspect of the femoral head and to reduce the flexion effect caused by the oblique plane osteotomy.[42]
4. Do not derotate the femur because this leads to an externally rotated gait similar to a femur fracture that heals in an externally rotated position.[43]
5. Medially translate the distal fragment to avoid developmental genu valgum.[44] To do this properly, a fixation implant that allows medialization of the femoral shaft should be used.
6. Perform trochanteric apophysiodesis to reduce trochanteric prominence.[40,44,45]
7. When the patient is 8 years or older and 20° of varus is required to contain the hip, then consider a limited amount of varus combined

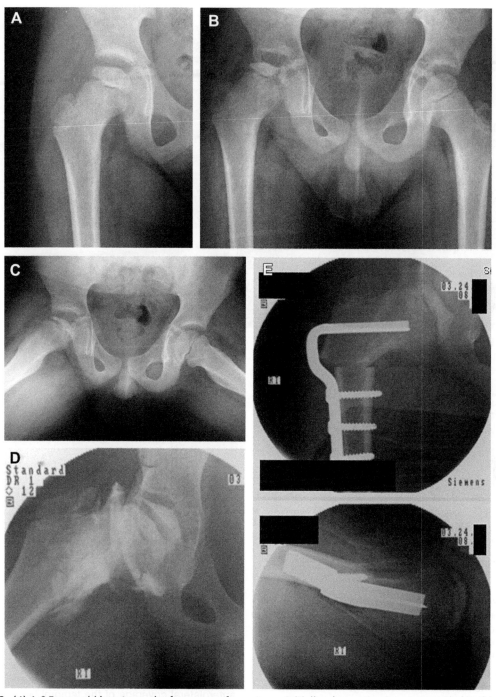

Fig. 3. (*A*) A 6.5-year-old boy 1 month after onset of symptoms. Initially, observation is recommended in this age group. (*B, C*) Radiographs 6 months after presentation show fragmentation stage of disease with progressive lateral migration with loss of height of the femoral head. (*D*) Arthrogram demonstrates containment without hinge abduction. Note deformity of femoral head even though it can still be contained. (*E*) Intraoperative radiographs show excessive varus with neck-shaft angle less than 115°. The patient was immobilized in a hip spica cast for 4 weeks. (*F*) Scanogram 1 year postoperative (8 years 1 month) demonstrates persistent varus with 2-cm limb-length discrepancy. (*G*) Scanogram at age 11 years demonstrates less than 1-cm limb-length discrepancy. (*H, I*) Anteroposterior (AP) radiograph standing and lateral radiograph at 14 years of age demonstrate Stulberg 2 outcome with spherical femoral head and improvement in articulo-trochanteric distance. Clinical examination demonstrated a normal gait, negative Trendelenburg test, and loss of 30° internal rotation and 20° of abduction compared with the opposite hip.

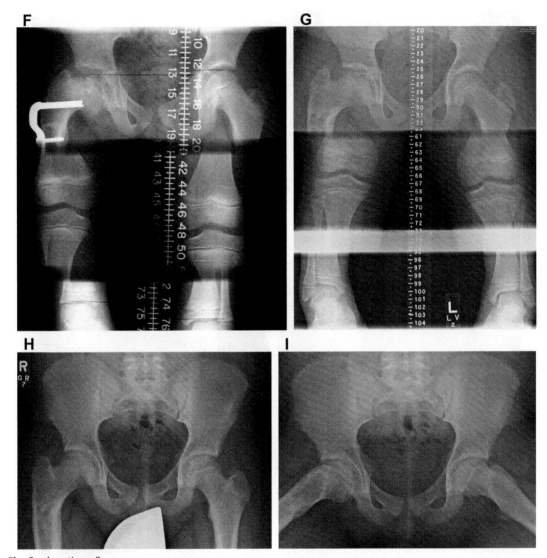

Fig. 3. (*continued*)

with a Salter osteotomy, pelvic rotational osteotomy, or shelf procedure to provide additional containment.[46] Combined osteotomies will avoid remodeling concerns in the older child. Triple innominate osteotomy may provide greater containment of the femoral head than Salter innominate osteotomy.

8. Postoperative immobilization may be unnecessary if excellent range of motion is restored before surgery.[47] When the osteotomy is performed without preliminary restoration of motion, postoperative immobilization in a spica cast is recommended for 4 to 6 weeks to allow resolution of muscle spasm.[19,39]

9. Avoid excessive abduction in a postoperative cast (if used) because this may contribute to avascular necrosis and growth disturbance.[48]

Containment by Salter Osteotomy

The Salter osteotomy is a transverse osteotomy of the pelvis along a line from the sciatic notch to just above the anterior inferior iliac spine. The acetabulum is then rotated laterally and anteriorly using the pubic symphysis as a hinge. This improves anterolateral coverage of the femoral head in the area most commonly affected in Perthes disease. The rotation of the osteotomy also displaces the acetabulum medially and increases the lever arm of the abductor muscles, thereby reducing the abductor force required to stabilize the hip.[49]

Salter reported improved outcomes following this osteotomy for Perthes disease compared with a group of similar untreated control patients.[1] Other investigators have also reported improved outcomes following a Salter osteotomy.[50,51] Investigators who compared innominate osteotomy to proximal femoral osteotomy found similar outcomes when appropriate treatment principles were followed.[3,52]

The authors consider the Salter osteotomy a useful form of containment for Perthes disease when patients are properly selected and the procedure is performed correctly. The most important considerations are to perform the procedure while the femoral head is round or almost round and to obtain a full or almost full range of motion before surgery.[5,50] Stevens and colleagues[50] advised that the osteotomy should be performed within 8 months of onset of symptoms. When a 30° wedge of bone is inserted anterolaterally, the anterior coverage of the femoral head can be improved by approximately 25° and lateral coverage of the femoral head by approximately 15°.[26,53]

Additional technical considerations include the following:

1. Residual contractures of the adductor muscle are released by subcutaneous tenotomy.[5]
2. An essential component of the procedure is to release the tendinous portion of the psoas muscle at the pelvic brim.[5,54]
3. The proximal or iliac segment should be stabilized so the movement occurs through the acetabular segment by rotation at the symphysis pubis.[54]
4. The osteotomy should remain closed posteriorly.[54]
5. Placing the involved lower extremity in the position can facilitate opening the osteotomy site in the correct orientation.[5]
6. The distal fragment should be displaced anteriorly approximately 1.0 to 1.5 cm to allow maximum pubic symphysis rotation and provide anterior coverage of the femoral head.[26]
7. A triangle of bone approximately 30° to 35° in shape is secured in the osteotomy site with 2 to 3 large threaded Steinmann pins.[26]
8. The Steinmann pins should be large enough to provide stability and avoid breakage.[54]
9. A postoperative cast is not required when the child is 6 years or older and can cooperate with toe-touch weight bearing for 4 to 6 weeks postoperatively.[5,26]
10. The Steinmann pins are removed 8 to 10 weeks postoperatively.

Containment by Shelf Procedures

Shelf acetabuloplasty is a procedure where the margin of the acetabulum is extended to provide more coverage for the femoral head. This increases the weight-bearing surface of the anterior, lateral, and/or posterior portions of the acetabulum. Shelf procedures do not change the orientation of the acetabulum so there is no change in the biomechanics of the hip except for the increased distribution of forces from the enlarged surface area. The Chiari osteotomy has some similarity to shelf procedures because it also increases the area of support for the femoral head. However, the Chiari osteotomy displaces the hip medially and superiorly and reduces the compression forces acting across the hip joint. The interposed capsule undergoes fibrous metaplasia and transforms into fibrocartilaginous tissue.[55] Although the Chiari osteotomy has been used for containment to prevent femoral head deformation,[56] it has primarily been recommended as a salvage procedure for advanced Perthes disease when the femoral head is extruded or incongruent.[57,58]

Several investigators have reported improved outcomes with containment by shelf acetabuloplasty.[59–62] Improved outcomes have also been reported with shelf acetabuloplasty for more advanced cases of Perthes disease with containable subluxation, and in patients 9 years and older.[59,63,64] One advantage of the shelf acetabuloplasty is preservation of limb length without excessive trochanteric prominence.[61,65] Another advantage is long-term improved coverage of the enlarged femoral head that develops following Perthes disease.[61,66,67] In children 8 years and older at time of shelf acetabuloplasty, the shelf is gradually incorporated into the growing pelvis without restricting range of motion at skeletal maturity.[60,62] This procedure can also be performed in children as young as 5 years without interfering with growth of the lateral acetabular margin.[62]

The authors consider shelf acetabuloplasty a useful form of containment for Perthes disease when patients are properly selected and the procedure is performed correctly. The bone graft should be placed in close contact with the joint capsule with sufficient autologous bone graft to buttress the extended margin of the acetabulum. The authors prefer the slotted acetabular augmentation described by Staheli and Chew.[68] In this procedure, the reflected head of the rectus femoris is dissected and left attached posteriorly. The capsule is thinned and cleared of all tissue. Using radiographic imaging, a narrow slot is created just proximal to the labrum. This slot is expanded anterolaterally and posterolaterally and then deepened in an oblique upward direction of approximately 15°. The cortical strips from the iliac crest are inserted into the slot. A properly developed slot will firmly hold the strips in place directly against the hip capsule and protrude far enough to establish a center-edge angle of approximately 45°.[68] The reflected head of the rectus femoris is sutured over the top of the cortical strips to hold them firmly against the hip capsule. The outer table of the ilium is elevated proximal to the slot without damaging the slot. Copious cancellous bone is packed against the lateral ilium proximal to the cortical strips that form the shelf. This provides a buttress of bone to support the shelf. A postoperative spica cast is not always necessary if the graft is secure and the child is cooperative with toe-touch weight bearing.[59,69]

Additional technical considerations include the following:

1. Place the graft near the joint line but above the growth area of the labral rim. Superiorly placed grafts tend to resorb.[69]
2. Avoid penetration of the joint while preparing the slot. A sufficiently oblique upward angle will prevent this and also ensure proper positioning of the cortical strips.[69]
3. The breadth of the slot from anterior to posterior should follow the curve of the capsule and should be sufficiently long to provide anterior, posterior, and lateral coverage.[68]

Containment by the Triple Pelvic Osteotomy

The triple pelvic osteotomy combines the transverse osteotomy of Salter with complete osteotomies of the superior pubic ramus and ischium (**Fig. 4**). This allows greater mobility of the acetabulum without interfering with growth of the triradiate cartilage. When a section of bone is removed from the ischium, or when the ischial and pubic osteotomies are close to the acetabulum, the acetabular fragment can be medialized to reduce the joint reaction forces.[70,71]

Use of the triple pelvic osteotomy has been proposed as a method of containment for older patients with more severe disease (**Fig. 5**).[72,73] Successful outcomes have been reported in hips with lateral migration and lateral pillar collapse (Herring C), as long as the hips were containable without hinge abduction.[71,72,74] However, outcomes of lateral pillar C cases have not been as satisfactory after the age of 8 years.[72]

The triple pelvic osteotomy can be used in any age group and provides greater containment than either the proximal femoral varus or Salter osteotomy alone.[71,72] Proximal femoral varus osteotomy is less likely to remodel after the age of 8 years[28,35] and Salter osteotomy may not provide adequate coverage in more severe cases or when femoral head flattening is present. Alternatives for containment in older children or more advanced cases with early femoral head flattening include triple pelvic osteotomy, shelf acetabuloplasty, or combined femoral and Salter osteotomy. Huang and Huang[75] compared shelf acetabuloplasty to triple pelvic osteotomy.[75] They found that outcomes were improved in both groups. The triple pelvic osteotomy was technically more demanding with more complications but the shelf augmentation group had fewer spherical hips at follow-up in a slightly older age group at time of surgery.

The authors consider triple pelvic osteotomy a useful form of containment for Perthes disease

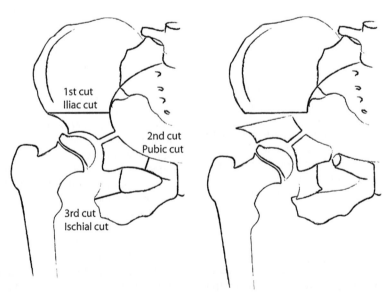

Fig. 4. Triple pelvic osteotomy allows greater mobility of the acetabulum and may allow greater coverage for advanced cases or older patients before onset of hinge abduction.

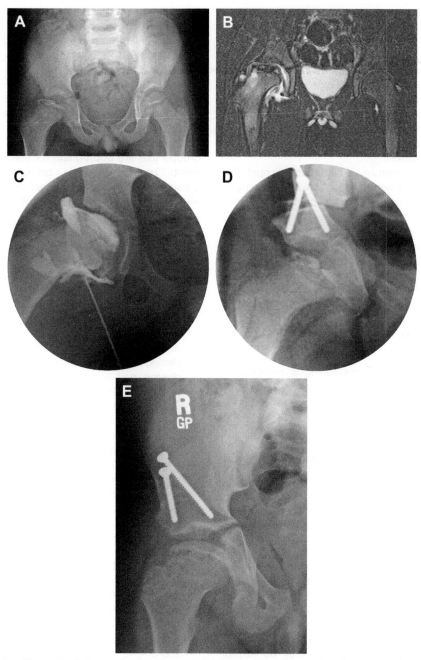

Fig. 5. (*A*) AP radiograph of the pelvis of an 8-year, 10-month-old boy 8 months after onset of Perthes disease. Note lateral migration with loss of containment of the femoral head. (*B*) Magnetic resonance image study confirms loss of containment and flattening of the femoral head with extrusion. The labrum is pushed upward by the enlarged, deformed femoral head. (*C*) Intraoperative arthrogram demonstrated near-containment. The supero-medial dye pool indicated marked deformity (flattening) of the femoral head. The labrum is compressed with abduction of the hip. (*D*) Intraoperative radiograph following triple pelvic osteotomy. Note that the lateral femoral head is now contained within the lateral margin of the acetabulum. (*E*) Radiography 16 months following triple pelvic osteotomy. Note the spherical, contained femoral head without acetabular deformity.

when patients are properly selected and the procedure is performed correctly. Additional training and experience may be needed to master the technique of triple pelvic osteotomy when compared with other methods of containment. The osteotomies are made close to the acetabulum, as described by Tonnis and colleagues,[76] but the osteotomies can generally be made through 2 separate incisions.[72,73] The iliac osteotomy is performed through a standard oblique anterolateral incision.

The pubic osteotomy is also made through the anterolateral incision but the ischial osteotomy is performed through a separate posterior incision. Other modifications have been described also, including a single anterolateral incision where the Ganz osteotome is used to complete the ischial cut using fluoroscopic guidance.[71,74,77] After the bone is cut, a bone clamp, threaded screw, or heavy threaded pin is used to rotate the acetabular fragment into the proper position. It is then fixed in position with cannulated screws.[70–72,77]

Additional technical considerations include the following:

1. Correct acetabular positioning is essential to avoid retroversion and excessive external rotation of the lower extremity.[78]
2. Avoid excessive containment that could cause impingement.[72]
3. A reconstruction plate may be used to stabilize the pubic osteotomy and reduce the risk of nonunion.[72,79]
4. A spica cast is unnecessary when stable fixation has been achieved.[72,73,77]

SUMMARY

Successful containment can be achieved by a variety of methods as long as the indications are correct and the method is followed according to recommended technique. Containment is generally unsuccessful when hinge abduction is present in the late fragmentation stage. Bed rest and range of motion treatment may be helpful before definitive containment but these are not considered containment methods at the present time. Cast or brace immobilization that includes the knees and limits weight bearing may be a successful method of containment, especially in children 6 to 8 years old; however, this requires a prolonged period of treatment.

Surgical containment allows return to full weight bearing and light activities approximately 8 weeks after surgery for most patients. Surgical containment is recommended as soon as the diagnosis is made in all children older than 8 years at onset. Proximal femoral varus osteotomy with trochanteric epiphysiodesis is primarily useful in children younger than 8 years because remodeling can result in equal leg lengths without excessive trochanteric prominence. Salter innominate osteotomy is also successful in this age group when the femoral head is round and almost full range of motion can be recovered preoperatively. Shelf augmentation is a widely accepted method of containment in all age groups that are appropriate for surgical containment. Triple innominate osteotomy provides greater containment than most other methods. All methods of containment are ill advised in the presence of hinge abduction.

REFERENCES

1. Salter RB. Legg-Calve-Perthes disease: the scientific basis for the methods of treatment and their indications. Clin Orthop Relat Res 1980;150:8–11.
2. Joseph B, Nair NS, Narashima Rao KL, et al. Optimal timing for containment surgery for Perthes disease. J Pediatr Orthop 2003;23:601–6.
3. Herring J, Kim MT, Browne R. Legg-Calve-Perthes disease: part II: prospective multicenter study of the effect of treatment on outcome. J Bone Joint Surg Am 2004;86:2121–34.
4. Ippolito E, Tudisco C, Farsetti P. The long-term prognosis of unilateral Perthes' disease. J Bone Joint Surg Br 1987;69:243–50.
5. Salter RB. Current concepts review: the present status of surgical treatment for Legg-Perthes disease. J Bone Joint Surg Am 1984;66:961–6.
6. Rosenfeld SB, Herring JA, Chao JC. Legg-Calve-Perthes disease: a review of cases with onset before six years of age. J Bone Joint Surg Am 2007;89(12):2712–22.
7. Canavese F, Dimeglio A. Perthes' disease: prognosis in children under six years of age. J Bone Joint Surg Br 2008;90(7):940–5.
8. Green NH, Beauchamp RD, Griffin PP. Epiphyseal extrusion as a prognostic indes in Legg-Calve-Perthes Disease. J Bone Joint Surg Am 1981;63:900–5.
9. Lappin K, Kealey D, Cosgrove A. Herring classification: how useful is the initial radiograph? J Pediatr Orthop 2002;22:479–82.
10. Carney BT, Minter CL. Nonsurgical treatment to regain hip abduction motion in Perthes disease: a retrospective review. South Med J 2004;97(5):485–8.
11. Wiig O, Terjesen T, Svenningsen S. Prognostic factors and outcome of treatment in Perthes' disease. J Bone Joint Surg Br 2008;90:1364–71.
12. Brech GC, Guarnieiro R. Evaluaton of physiotherapy in the treatment of Legg-Calve-Perthes Disease. Clinics (Sao Paulo) 2006;61(6):521–8.

13. Terjesen T, Wiig O, Svenningsen S. The natural history of Perthes' disease. Acta Orthop 2010; 81(6):708–14.

14. Stanitski CL. Hip range of motion in Perthes' disease: comparison of pre-operative and intra-operative values. J Child Orthop 2007;1(1):33–5.

15. Brotherton BJ, McKibbin B. Perthes' disease treated by prolonged recumbency and femoral head containment: a long-term appraisal. J Bone Joint Surg Br 1977;59:8–14.

16. Petrie JG, Bitenc I. The abduction weight-bearing treatment in Legg-Perthes' disease. J Bone Joint Surg Br 1971;53(1):54–62.

17. Kiepurska A. Late results of treatment in Perthes' disease by a functional method. Clin Orthop Relat Res 1991;272:76–81.

18. Rab GT, Wyatt M, Sutherland DH, et al. A technique for determining femoral head containment during gait. J Pediatr Orthop 1985;5:8–12.

19. Thompson GH, Westin GW. Legg-Calve-Perthes disease: results of discontinuing treatment in the early reossification phase. Clin Orthop Relat Res 1979;139:70–80.

20. Price CT, Day DD, Flynn JC. Behavioral sequelae of bracing versus surgery for Legg-Calve-Perthes disease. J Pediatr Orthop 1988;8:285–7.

21. Meehan PL, Angel D, Nelson JM. The Scottish Rite abduction orthosis in the treatment of Legg-Perthes Disease. J Bone Joint Surg Am 1992;74:2–12.

22. Martinez AG, Weinstein SL, Dietz FR. The weight-bearing abduction brace for the treatment of Legg-Perthes disease. J Bone Joint Surg Am 1992;74:12–21.

23. Aksoy MC, Caglar O, Yazici M, et al. Comparison between braced and non-braced Legg-Calve-Perthes-disease patients: a radiological outcome study. J Pediatr Orthop B 2004;13:153–7.

24. Savvidis E, Loer F. Ein behandlungsprinzip mit fragwurdiger wirksamkeit bei morbus Perthes. Z Orthop Ihre Grenzgeb 1992;130:120–4 [in German].

25. Menelaus MB. Lessons learned in the management of Legg-Calve-Perthes disease. Clin Orthop Relat Res 1986;209:41–8.

26. Thompson GH, Price CT, Roy D, et al. Legg-Calve-Perthes disease: current concepts. Instr Course Lect 2002;51:367–84.

27. Axer A. Subtrochanteric osteotomy in the treatment of Perthes' disease. J Bone Joint Surg Br 1965;47:489–99.

28. Leitch JM, Paterson DC, Foster BK. Growth disturbance in Legg-Calve-Perthes disease and consequences of surgical treatment. Clin Orthop Relat Res 1991;262:178–84.

29. Hoikka V, Poussa M, Yrjonen T, et al. Intertrochanteric varus osteotomy for Perthes' disease: radiographic changes after 2–16-year follow-up of 126 hips. Acta Orthop Scand 1991;62:549–53.

30. Noonan KJ, Price CT, Kupiszewski SJ, et al. Results of femoral varus osteotomy in children older than 9 years of age with Perthes disease. J Pediatr Orthop 2001;21:198–204.

31. Maquet P. Biomechanics of hip dysplasia. Acta Orthop Belg 1999;65(3):302–14.

32. Iwasaki K. The change in venous circulation of the proximal part of the femur after varus osteotomy in Perthes' disease. Nippon Seikeigeka Gakkai Zasshi 1986;60:237–49.

33. Marklund T, Tillberg B. Coxa plana: a radiological comparison of the rate of healing with conservative measures and after osteotomy. J Bone Joint Surg Br 1976;58:25–30.

34. Joseph B, Narashima R, Mulpuri K, et al. How does a femoral varus osteotomy alter the natural evolution of Perthes' disease? J Pediatr Orthop B 2005;14:10–5.

35. Mirovsky Y, Axer A, Hendel D. Residual shortening after osteotomy for Perthes' disease. J Bone Joint Surg Br 1984;66:184–8.

36. Axer A, Gershuni DH, Hendel D, et al. Indications for femoral osteotomy in Legg-Calve-Perthes disease. Clin Orthop Relat Res 1980;150:78–87.

37. Canario AT, Williams L, Weintroub S, et al. A controlled study of the results of femoral osteotomy in severe Perthes' disease. J Bone Joint Surg Br 1980;62:438–40.

38. Bowen JR, Schreiber FC, Foster BK, et al. Premature femoral neck physical closure in Perthes' disease. Clin Orthop Relat Res 1982;171:24–9.

39. Lloyd-Roberts GC, Catterall A, Salamon PB. A controlled study of the indications for and the results of femoral osteotomy in Perthes' disease. J Bone Joint Surg Br 1976;58:31–6.

40. Weiner SD, Weiner DS, Riley PM. Pitfalls in treatment of Legg-Calve-Perthes disease using proximal femoral varus osteotomy. J Pediatr Orthop 1991;11:20–4.

41. Kim H, da Cunha AM, Browne R, et al. How much varus is optimal with proximal femoral osteotomy to preserve the femoral head in Legg-Calvé-Perthes disease? J Bone Joint Surg Am 2011;93:341–7.

42. Bayliss N, Margetts M, Taylor JF. Intertrochanteric femoral osteotomy for Legg-Calve-Perthes' disease. J Pediatr Orthop B 1994;3:15–7.

43. Hansson G, Wallin J. External rotational positioning of the leg after intertrochanteric combined varus-derotational osteotomy in Perthes' disease. Arch Orthop Trauma Surg 1997;116:108–11.

44. Kitakoji T, Hattori T, Iwata H. Femoral varus osteotomy in Legg-Calve-Perthes disease: points at operation to prevent residual problems. J Pediatr Orthop 1999;19:76–81.

45. Shah H, Siddesh ND, Joseph B, et al. Effect of prophylactic trochanteric epiphyseodesis in older children with Perthes' disease. J Pediatr Orthop 2009;29(8):889–95.

46. Crutcher JP, Staheli LT. Combined osteotomy as a salvage procedure for severe Legg-Calve-Perthes disease. J Pediatr Orthop 1992;12:151–6.

47. Joseph B, Srinivas G, Thomas R. Management of Perthes disease of late onset in Southern India. J Bone Joint Surg Br 1996;78:625–30.

48. Barnes JM. Premature epiphyseal closure in Perthes' disease. J Bone Joint Surg Br 1980;62:432–7.

49. Rab GT. Biomechanical aspects of the Salter osteotomy. Clin Orthop Relat Res 1978;132:82–7.

50. Stevens PM, Williams P, Menelaus M. Innominate osteotomy for Perthes' disease. J Pediatr Orthop 1981;1(1):47–54.

51. Paterson DC, Leitch JM, Foster BK, Results of innominate osteotomy in the treatment of Legg-Calve-Perthes disease. Clin Orthop Relat Res 1991;266:96–103.

52. Sponseller PD, Desai SS, Millis MB. Comparison of femoral and innominate osteotomies for the treatment of Legg-Calve-Perthes disease. J Bone Joint Surg Am 1988;70:1131–9.

53. Rab GT. Containment of the hip: a theoretical comparison of osteotomies. Clin Orthop Relat Res 1981;154:191–6.

54. Salter RB. Specific guidelines in the application of the principle of innominate osteotomy. Orthop Clin North Am 1972;3(1):149–56.

55. Hiranuma S, Higuchi F, Inoue A, et al. Changes in the interposed capsule after Chiari osteotomy. J Bone Joint Surg Br 1992;74(3):463–7.

56. Cahuzac JP, Onimus M, Trottmann F, et al. Chiari pelvic osteotomy in Perthes' disease. J Pediatr Orthop 1990;10:163–6.

57. Redddy RR, Morin C. Chiari osteotomy in Legg-Calve-Perthes disease. J Pediatr Orthop B 2005;14:1–9.

58. Bennett JT, Mazurek RT, Cash JD. Chiari's osteotomy in the treatment of Perthes' disease. J Bone Joint Surg Br 1991;73:225–8.

59. Yoo WJ, Choi IH, Cho T-J, et al. Shelf acetabuloplasty for children with Perthes' disease and reducible subluxation of the hip. J Bone Joint Surg Br 2009;91(10):1383–7.

60. Daly K, Bruce C, Catterall A. Lateral shelf acetabuloplasty in Perthes' disease. J Bone Joint Surg Br 1999;81:380–4.

61. Willett K, Hudson I, Catterall A. Lateral shelf acetabuloplasty: an operation for older children with Perthes' disease. J Pediatr Orthop 1992;12:563–8.

62. Jacobs R, Moens P, Fabry G. Lateral shelf acetabuloplasty in the early stage of Legg-Calve-Perthes disease with special emphasis on the remaining growth of the acetabulum: a preliminary report. J Pediatr Orthop B 2004;13:21–8.

63. Dimitriou JK, Leonidou O, Pettas N. Acetabulum augmentation for Legg-Calve-Perthes disease. Acta Orthop Scand Suppl 1997;275:103–5.

64. Kruse RW, Guille JT, Bowen JR. Shelf arthroplasty in patients who have Legg-Calve-Perthes disease. J Bone Joint Surg Am 1991;73:1338–47.

65. Grzegorzewski A, Synder M, Kozlowski P, et al. Leg length discrepancy in Legg-Calve-Perthes disease. J Pediatr Orthop 2005;25(2):206–9.

66. Domzalski ME, Glutting J, Bowen JR, et al. Lateral acetabular growth stimulation following a labral support procedure in Legg-Calve-Perthes disease. J Bone Joint Surg Am 2006;88(7):1458–66.

67. Grzegorzewski A, Synder M, Kozlowski P, et al. The role of the acetabulum in Perthes' disease. J Pediatr Orthop 2006;26(3):316–21.

68. Staheli LT, Chew DE. Slotted acetabular augmentation in childhood and adolescence. J Pediatr Orthop 1992;12(5):560 80.

69. Crawford AH, Herrera-Soto JA. Shelf acetabuloplasty of the hip. In: Tolo VT, Skaggs DL, editors. Master techniques in orthopedic surgery: pediatrics. Philadelphia: Wolters Kluwer/Lippincott Williams & Wilkins; 2008. p. 165–73.

70. Lipton GE, Bowen JR. A new modified technique of triple osteotomy of the innominate bone for acetabular dysplasia. Clin Orthop Relat Res 2005;434:78–85.

71. Kumar D, Bache CE, O'Hara JN. Interlocking triple pelvic osteotomy in severe Legg-Calve-Perthes disease. J Pediatr Orthop 2002;22:464–70.

72. Wenger DR, Pring ME, Hosalker HS, et al. Advanced containment methods for Legg-Calve-Perthes disease: results of triple pelvic osteotomy. J Pediatr Orthop 2010;30:749–57.

73. Vukasinovic Z, Spasovski D, Vucetic C, et al. Triple pelvic osteotomy in the treatment of Legg-Calve-Perthes disease. Int Orthop 2009;33:1377–83.

74. Conroy E, Sheehan E, O'Connor P, et al. Triple pelvic osteotomy in Legg-Calve-Perthes disease using a single anterolateral incision: a 4-year review. J Pediatr Orthop B 2010;19:323–6.

75. Huang MJ, Huang SC. Surgical treatment of severe Perthes disease: comparison of triple osteotomy and shelf augmentation. J Formos Med Assoc 1999;98(3):183–9.

76. Tonnis D, Behrens K, Tscharani F. A modified technique of the triple pelvic osteotomy: early results. J Pediatr Orthop 1981;1:241–9.

77. O'Connor PA, Mulhall KJ, Kearns SR, et al. Triple pelvic osteotomy in Legg-Calve-Perthes disease using a single anterolateral incision. J Pediatr Orthop B 2003;12:387–9.

78. Frick SL, Kim SS, Wenger DR. Pre- and postoperative three-dimensional computed tomography analysis of triple innominate osteotomy for hip dysplasia. J Pediatr Orthop 2000;20(1):116–23.

79. Tonnis D. Pelvic operations for dysplasia of the hip. In: Tonnis D, editor. Congenital dysplasia and dislocation of the hip in children and adults. Heidelberg (Germany): Springer-Verlag; 1987. p. 370–81.

Principles of Treatment in Late Stages of Perthes Disease

In Ho Choi, MD*, Won Joon Yoo, MD, Tae-Joon Cho, MD,
Hyuk Ju Moon, MD

KEYWORDS
• Principle of treatment • Late stage • Perthes disease

Some children with severe Legg-Calvé-Perthes disease (LCPD; Catterall 3 or 4, Herring B/C or C), may present late in the course of the disease, that is, in late fragmentation or reossification stage, with an already collapsed and deformed femoral head due to undue force passing through the anterosuperolateral aspect of the femoral head. Abnormal hinge movement of the hip joint, so-called hinge abduction, is the result of extrusion of the epiphyseal segment of the femoral head. If hinge abduction is fixed, abnormal hinge movement results in progressive subluxation, collapse of lateral pillar, and widening of the femoral head, preventing it sliding into the acetabular socket completely.[1–6] The resulting alteration in the center of rotation presents with restricted hip motion, which is often associated with antalgic gait, short-limb gait, Trendelenburg gait, Duchenne gait, and out-toeing or in-toeing gaits. The authors reported that out-toeing and in-toeing gaits are apparently caused by the compensatory rotation of the proximal femur to avoid impingement by placing the femoral hump to the relatively deficient anterolateral part of the hip joint.[7]

It is of paramount importance to distinguish hips that may or may not be suitable for containment in the transitional stage, because long-term clinical and radiological outcomes may be influenced by the choice of treatment. This article summarizes the definition of hinge abduction, pathoanatomy of hinge segment, assessment of hinge abduction, determination of reducible and irreducible hinge abduction, and treatment strategies for containable and uncontainable hips in the transitional stage (fragmentation to early reossification stage).

DEFINITION OF HINGE ABDUCTION

Hinge abduction was first described by Grossbard,[8] who described abnormal hinge movement in 4 patients with residual deformity in LCPD. The concept of hinge abduction was further elucidated by Catterall,[3,4] who demonstrated the value of intraoperative arthrography in determining the presence of abnormal hinge movement. These authors defined, using intraoperative dynamic arthrography, that hinge abduction is a phenomenon of impingement of the outer part of the femoral head onto the lateral lip of the acetabulum, typically showing widening of medial joint space by levering the inferomedial portion of the femoral head laterally away from the teardrop in the acetabular floor in abduction on the anteroposterior (AP) view. Nakamura and colleagues[9] further refined the definition of hinge abduction to include the observance of an increasing subluxation index (percentage ratio of the medial joint space to the acetabular width) with abduction or a positive impingement sign. They defined the latter as the relationship of the tangential point of the most superior part of

No benefits in any form have been received or will be received from any commercial party related directly or indirectly to the subject of this article.
Division of Pediatric Orthopaedics, Seoul National University Children's Hospital, 101 Daehak-ro, Jongno-gu, 110-744 Seoul, Korea
* Corresponding author.
E-mail address: inhoc@snu.ac.kr

epiphysis to the lateral edge of the bony acetabular rim in maximum abduction.

PATHOANATOMY OF HINGE SEGMENT AND ASSESSMENT OF HINGE ABDUCTION

The collapse and subluxation of the femoral head appear to be influenced differently by area of necrosis, mechanical properties of the necrotic segment, and direction of hip loading force in severely involved LCPD.[10] Rab and colleagues[10] demonstrated in a theoretical study on subluxation using a 3-dimensional rigid body spring method hip model that the direction of subluxation was sensitive to the direction of hip loading force, which might be modified by the presence of pain and contractures. Three-dimensional pathoanatomy of the hinge segment may differ in each patient, and thereby the pattern of abnormal hinge movement can vary according to the size, location, and configuration of the impinging hump.[6] Pécasse and colleagues[11] claimed that deformation of the femoral head is usually multidirectional, flat, or broad in the frontal pane and phalloid in the axial direction. The authors have observed that the main hump on the femoral head can locate from anterior to lateral aspect of the femoral head.[6] In this context, the authors think that hinge abduction is a complex manifestation of the hinge movement occurring in the continuum between lateral and anterior impingement.[6,7]

The earliest clinical sign of abnormal hinge movement during follow-up, in general, is a sudden deterioration in range of motion of the hip, particularly abduction. When diagnosis of hinge abduction is suspected, the nature of the abnormal hinge movement should be carefully evaluated. It is essential to examine the hip to see whether it is caused either by contractures of adductor muscles or by true hinge abduction due to impingement of the deformed head against acetabular rim.[1]

Three-dimensional understanding of hinge movement is important in planning the surgical method, because the pattern of abnormal hinge movement can vary according to the spatial features of the impinging hump of the femoral head. Preoperatively, the authors usually take plain AP radiographs with the hip in neutral, abduction, adduction, and frog-leg lateral position in addition to false profile view to determine subluxation and congruity. The authors found that 3-dimensional computed tomography (CT) examination with multiplanar reformation images is useful to assess the spatial features of the hinge segment of the femoral head. Magnetic resonance (MR) and ultrasound images also provide valuable information about spatial features of osteocartilaginous hinge segment.

Intraoperatively, dynamic arthrography under general anesthesia is very helpful to determine the position of stability and congruity between the femoral head and the acetabulum. Lateral impingement can be detected on the anteroposterior arthrograms of the hip by moving the lower limb in adduction/abduction in combination with the internal rotation/external rotation position. In contrast, anterior impingement[5,6] can be checked in the true lateral arthrograms of the hip by moving the hip into the flexion/extension position. The congruent position of the superior portion of the head is also confirmed by taking the craniocaudal projection of the image with the hip in extension.[6]

DETERMINATION OF REDUCIBLE AND IRREDUCIBLE HINGE ABDUCTION

With hinge abduction, the center of movement of the femoral head is located on the lateral edge of acetabulum, and the labrum is deformed upwards in attempted abduction. Reducible hinge abduction can be demonstrated by the position of the femoral head that would center within the acetabulum in abduction without imposing undue pressure on the lateral edge of the acetabulum.[6,12,13] The authors think that Hilgenreiner–labral angle[13] and epiphyseal slip-in index[14] measured in abduction on anteroposterior view of the arthrograms provide an objective measure of the degree of reducibility of flattened and extruded femoral head underneath the acetabulum (**Fig. 1**). Hilgenreiner–labral angle is defined as the angle between the line parallel to the Hilgenreiner line and the line connecting the lateral acetabular margin and the labral tip in abduction between 30° and 45°.[13] Epiphyseal slip-in index is calculated as the horizontal distance from lateral margin of the bony acetabular rim to the tip (tangential point) of the epiphysis slipping into the acetabulum in 40° of abduction relative to the horizontal distance between the lateral margin of the bony acetabular rim and the tip of the tear drop (acetabular depth).[14] When there is irreducible hinge abduction, neither Hilgenreiner–labral angle nor epiphyseal slip-in index would substantially be improved in abduction.

TREATMENT STRATEGY FOR THE HIPS WITH REDUCIBLE HINGE ABDUCTION

In the transitional stage, if the epiphyseal collapse is not advanced, and the extruded epiphyseal segment is relatively small and soft enough to slip easily underneath the labrum on attempted abduction without imposing undue pressure on the lateral edge of the acetabulum, the hip can be deemed appropriate for containment. The authors' current

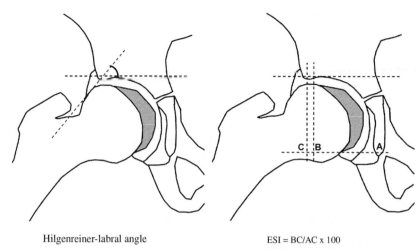

Hilgenreiner-labral angle   ESI = BC/AC x 100

Fig. 1. Hilgenreiner-labral angle *(left)* and Epiphyseal slip-in index (ESI) *(right)* Hilgenreiner–labral angle is defined as the angle between the line parallel to the Hilgenreiner line and the line connecting the lateral acetabular margin and the labral tip in abduction between 30° and 45°. Epiphyseal slip-in index, which is calculated as the horizontal distance from lateral margin of the bony acetabular rim to the tip (tangential point) of the epiphysis slipping into the acetabulum in 40° of abduction relative to the horizontal distance between the lateral margin of the bony acetabular rim and the tip of the tear drop (acetabular depth). (*Data from* Kamegaya M, Saisu T, Takazawa M, et al. Arthrographic indicators for decision making about femoral varus osteotomy in Legg-Calvé-Perthes disease. J Child Orthop 2008;2(4):261–7.)

treatment approach for hinge abduction when detected during the transitional stage is as follows. The patient is placed in bed rest for abduction traction for approximately 1 week, and then the patient is taken to the operating theater for arthrographic assessment under general anesthesia. If the hip has reducible hinge abduction, the authors prefer to perform soft tissue release via medial approach that includes adductor tenotomy and psoas tenotomy, with or without medial joint capsular release sequentially to achieve abduction beyond 45°. The patient is then placed in Petrie cast for 3 to 6 weeks to maintain the femoral head in the acetabulum. At the end of this period, appropriate surgical containment (eg, femoral varus osteotomy,[1,14] double-level osteotomy [**Fig. 2**],[15,16] triple innominate osteotomy,[17,18] and shelf acetabuloplasty [**Fig. 3**]),[12,13,19,20] is undertaken, taking into consideration of the age, femoral neck-shaft angle, and the extent of uncoverage of the femoral head. After bony healing, the patient continues a program of intensive physical and hydrotherapy with protective partial weight bearing and night-time abduction splintage for several months.

Containment treatment for reducible hinge abduction appears to be beneficial for younger children, because they have greatest remaining growth potential. Kamegaya and colleagues[14] reported that an epiphyseal slip-in index of 20% or more determined a safe zone for predicting an acceptable outcome (80% sensitivity, 89% specificity, and a 7.2 likelihood ratio) with femoral varus osteotomy that was performed in patients with an age of at least 8 years at onset and Herring class B or Catterall's 3 with subluxation or persistent limitation of the range of hip motion, or all ages with Herring class C or Catterall's 4 before the healing stage.

Shelf acetabuloplasty is believed to be beneficial for hip remodeling by preventing hip subluxation and stimulating lateral acetabular growth in the selected subgroup of hips in the fragmentation stage showing reducible hinge abduction.[13,20] The authors previously reported that only when a 'comfortable labrum (Hilgenreiner–labral angle >35°) was correlated with satisfactory hip remodeling with increased acetabular depth growth and the prevention of hip subluxation after shelf acetabuloplasty for children with reducible subluxation.[13] The authors agree with others that Salter innominate osteotomy or Pemberton osteotomy may not be indicated in older patients (older than 6 years old) with deformed femoral heads (more than 3 mm deviation from sphericity).[21,22] It is not only because of potential increase of the forces between the lateral aspect of the femoral head and acetabulum, but also because of difficulty to contain enlarged femoral head.

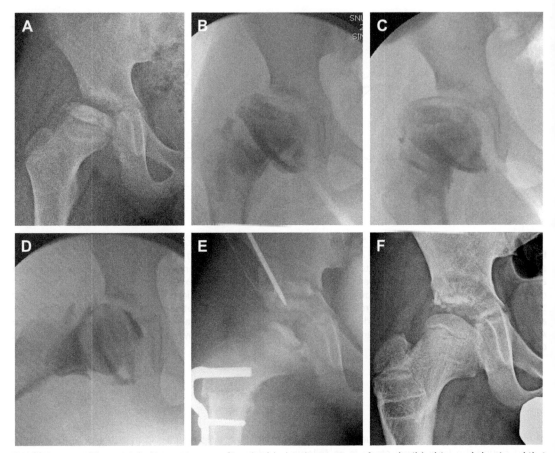

Fig. 2. A case with a satisfactory outcome after double-level osteotomy for reducible hinge abduction. (*A*) A radiograph of an 8-year-9 month-old boy shows subluxated femoral head in the fragmentation stage. An abduction cast with tenotomy of adductor and psoas was performed as an initial surgery. Arthrograms (*B–D*) at the time of femoral varus osteotomy and Dega osteotomy (*E*) suggest reducible hinge abduction; the labral position is assessed as uncomfortable (labral tip is at the same level with the tip of the epiphysis) in hip neutral (*B*) and adduction (*C*), but as comfortable (>35° of Hilgenreiner–labral angle) in abduction (*D*). (*F*) A radiograph taken 2 years after surgery shows a well-contained, round femoral head with Stulberg type 2 deformity.

TREATMENT STRATEGY FOR THE HIPS WITH IRREDUCIBLE HINGE ABDUCTION

When the child presents late with established hinge abduction due to enlarged, crushed femoral head, the hip may remain irreducible. On arthrograms, the labrum is usually further deformed upwards by the hinging segment of the femoral head in attempted abduction even after soft tissue release. In this situation, further attempts to contain the femoral head may be more harmful rather than helpful.[1,23] Hence, surgical treatment modality should be changed from one that depends upon remodeling by containment of the femoral head to the one that improves joint congruity and that reduces femoroacetabular impingement (FAI) by reducing nonphysiologic forces through the hip joint.[6,24] Several surgical techniques have been described

to address irreducible hinge abduction, including proximal femoral valgus osteotomy,[6,24,25] acetabular enlarging procedure,[13,22,26] hip joint distraction,[27–31] osteochondroplasty,[32] and femoral head reshaping procedure. The latter 2 methods may not be indicated for the hips with irreducible hinge abduction in the transitional stage.

The rationale for valgus osteotomy in the treatment of hinge abduction is to alleviate abnormal hinge movement and to realign the leg with the hip in the position of best fit in neutral weight-bearing position.[2–4,6,24,25] Although some authors reserve proximal femoral valgus osteotomy for healed Perthes disease,[25,26] the authors of this article think that valgus osteotomy should first be contemplated, regardless of the stage, if the femoral head and acetabulum become congruent when the joint is adducted but remain incongruent

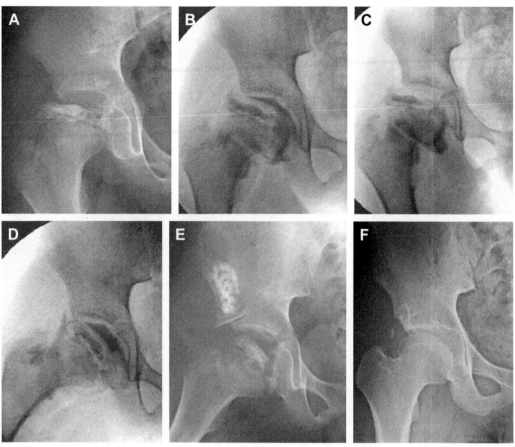

Fig. 3. A case with a satisfactory outcome after shelf acetabuloplasty for reducible hinge abduction. (*A*) A radiograph of an 8-year-4 month-old boy shows subluxated femoral head in the fragmentation stage. Arthrograms suggest reducible hinge abduction; the labral position is assessed as uncomfortable (labral tip is at the same level with the tip of the epiphysis) in hip neutral (*B*) and adduction (*C*), but as comfortable (>35° of Hilgenreiner-labral angle) in abduction (*D*). An abduction cast with tenotomy of adductor and psoas was followed by shelf acetabuloplasty (*E*). (*F*) A radiograph taken at 6 years and 10 months after surgery shows a round femoral head with Stulberg type 2 deformity, suggestive of satisfactory hip remodeling with increased acetabular depth growth and prevention of hip subluxation.

in a neutral or abducted position (**Fig. 4**).[6,24] This may be particularly true for the cases of severe late-onset LCPD that is diagnosed after 9 to 10 years of age, when epiphyseal collapse is rather rapid, and the healing process is prolonged with limited remodeling capacity.[23] Decision making as to whether the rotational/sagittal components would be combined with valgization should be based upon careful determination of the spatial features of the hump of the femoral head.[6] There is controversy as to whether the acetabular procedure, including innominate osteotomy, shelf acetabuloplasty, or Chiari osteotomy, should be performed simultaneously or as a second-stage procedure to cover the extruded femoral head at the time of a valgus osteotomy. The authors prefer to delay the acetabular procedures, particularly in the younger patient. This is

because an impinging hump can regress in size with time after operation in accordance with remodeling of the hip. This may enable a hyaline cartilage-to-hyaline cartilage redirectional acetabular osteotomy (eg, triple innominate osteotomy or periacetabular osteotomy) as a second-stage procedure, instead of a hyaline cartilage-to-fibrocartilage salvage procedure (eg, Chiari osteotomy or shelf acetabuloplasty), depending on the degree of roundness of the femoral head. However, if there is a substantial increase in subluxation and the hip remains unstable following a valgus osteotomy, a concomitant acetabular procedure is necessary to obtain adequate acetabular coverage, and thus decrease the unit load on the articular cartilage.[6]

Reports on the value of hip joint distraction started to appear in the literature in the early

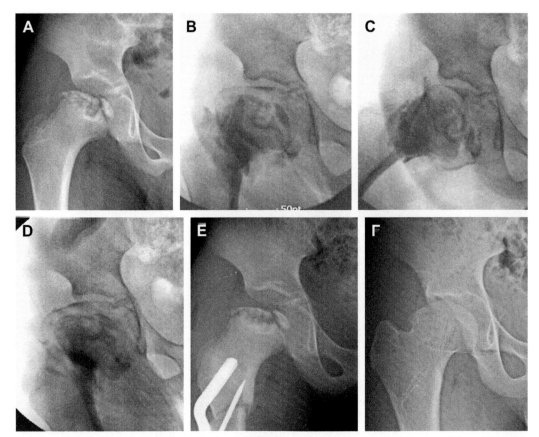

Fig. 4. A case treated by proximal femoral valgus osteotomy for irreducible hinge abduction. (*A*) A radiograph of a 7-year-4 month-old boy shows markedly collapsed, subluxated femoral head in the fragmentation stage. On arthrograms, the femoral head and acetabulum remain incongruent in a neutral (*B*) or abducted (*C*) position, but becomes congruent in adducted position (*D*). The labral position is assessed as uncomfortable (<35° of Hilgenreiner–labral angle; minus epiphyseal slip-in index) in abduction (*C*). A radiograph taken 7 years and 4 months after femoral valgus osteotomy (*E*) shows a congruent hip but with mildly ovoid femoral head, suggestive of Stulberg type 3 deformity (*F*). His hip function was near normal at the latest follow-up at age 15 years.

1990s.[27] The concept of articulated hip distraction combines off-loading of muscles and body forces with distraction of the joint space by means of an external fixator (EF) that crosses the hip joint. However, the indications and expected results of hip joint distraction are controversial and have yet to be fully documented.[27–31] Kocaoglu and colleagues[28] found overall poor results in children, with an average age of 7.5 years, treated by the nonarticulated Ilizarov fixator to distract the hip joint for less than 4 months. On the other hand, other reports using articulated, hip distraction, which enables maintaining the hip motion in the apparatus, have been favorable with short-term follow-up. Kukukkaya and colleagues[29] reported good results in terms of hip sphericity and joint congruity in 11 patients with avascular necrosis (8 patients with Perthes disease), who were treated by articulated, Ilizarov fixator for an average of 3.5 months.

Segev and colleagues[30] reported on, at a mean follow-up of 2 years 7 months, 16 children with severe late-onset LCPD surgically treated at average age of 12 years and 1 month (9 years 4 months to 15 years) by soft tissue release (tenotomy of adductor and psoas) and articulated hip distraction. Joint distraction with an articulated EF was used for 4 to 5 months until lateral pillar reossification appeared. They reported that an improvement of hip range of motion was found in all patients; additionally, the contour of the femoral head was improved. However, the Stulberg classifications on the last follow-up were type 3 for 3 hips and type 4 for the other 13 hips. They attributed a poor prognosis to their age and the severity of the disease at presentation.

In the authors' limited experience, soft tissue release and articulated hip distraction (4–6 months) in adolescents with severe LCPD in the transitional stage has resulted in reduced pain and limp, and a gain in range of hip motion, without significant change in the sphericity of the femoral head. However, the authors have experienced that pin loosening and incompliance to floxion–extension exercise were frequent and troublesome. Potential contamination of abductor muscles by pin track infection appears to be another concern for future total hip replacement. The authors, therefore, have a stance that articulated hip distraction should be selectively used only for the uncontainable, severely subluxated hips in adolescents or young adults, in whom other conventional methods have proven to be insufficient in providing containment. An additional indication would be when the hip remains stiff because of irreducible hinge abduction.

SUMMARY

Children with severely involved LCPD may present in late fragmentation stage or reossification stage, often associated with femoral head flattening and extrusion. This may result in hinge abduction, which appears to be a complex manifestation of the hinge movement occurring in the continuum between lateral and anterior impingement.

It is essential to distinguish hips that may or may not be suitable for containment in the transitional stage. If the arthrograms suggest reducible hinge abduction, various containment surgeries can be chosen, depending on the age, femoral neck-shaft angle, and extent of uncoverage of the femoral head, to eliminate FAI and to prevent further deformation of the femoral head. In contrast, if the hip has a severely deformed femoral head with irreducible hinge abduction, restoration of joint congruity and reduction of FAI should be the primary goals of treatment. Realignment by valgus osteotomy to the neutral position of weight bearing is the most commonly preferred procedure for the hips with irreducible subluxation in view of restoration of joint congruity and reduction of FAI. Valgus osteotomy, if necessary, combined with other acetabular procedures, has been proven to contribute to the sustained improvement of symptoms and function, and to beneficially influence remodeling of the hip. Articulated hip distraction appears to be an emerging modality, yet to be fully determined, in subgroup of late-presenting patients with stiff hips due to hinge abduction, in whom other conventional methods have proven to be insufficient. Positive clinical and radiological observations following aforementioned surgical treatments for the hips with advanced epiphyseal collapse and extrusion of the femoral do not preclude the possibility of the future development of degenerative arthritis in the adulthood.

REFERENCES

1. Reinker KA. Early diagnosis and treatment of hinge abduction in Legg-Perthes disease. J Pediatr Orthop 1990,10(1):3–9.
2. Raney EM, Grogan DP, Hurley ME, et al. The role of proximal femoral valgus osteotomy in Legg-Calvé-Perthes disease. Orthopedics 2002;25(5):513–7.
3. Quain S, Catterall A. Hinge abduction of the hip: diagnosis and treatment. J Bone Joint Surg 1986;68(1):61–4.
4. Catterall A. Legg-Calve-Perthes disease. Edinburgh (UK): Churchill Livingstone; 1982.
5. Snow SW, Keret D, Scarangella S, et al. Anterior impingement of the femoral head: a late phenomenon of Legg-Calvé-Perthes disease. J Pediatr Orthop 1993;13(3):286–9.
6. Yoo WJ, Choi IH, Chung CY, et al. Valgus femoral osteotomy for hinge abduction in Perthes disease: decision making and outcomes. J Bone Joint Surg 2004;86B(5):726–30.
7. Yoo WJ, Choi IH, Cho TJ, et al. Out-toeing and in-toeing in patients with Perthes disease: role of the femoral hump. J Pediatr Orthop 2008;28(7):717–22.
8. Grossbard GD. Hip pain during adolescence after Perthes disease. J Bone Joint Surg 1981;63B(4):572–4.
9. Nakamura J, Kamegaya M, Saisu T, et al. Hip arthrography under general anesthesia to refine the definition of hinge abduction in Legg-Calvé-Perthes disease. J Pediatr Orthop 2008;28(6):614–8.
10. Rab GT, Wyatt M, Sutherland DH, et al. A technique for determining femoral head containment during gait. J Pediatr Orthop 1985;5(1):8–12.
11. Pécasse GA, Eijer H, Haverkamp D, et al. Intertrochanteric osteotomy in young adults for sequelae of Legg-Calvé-Perthes disease—a long term follow-up. Int Orthop (SICOT) 2004;28(1):44–7.
12. Daly K, Bruce C, Catterall A. Lateral shelf acetabuloplasty in Perthes disease. A review of the end of growth. J Bone Joint Surg 1999;81B(3):380–4.
13. Yoo WJ, Choi IH, Cho TJ, et al. Shelf acetabuloplasty for children with Perthes disease and with reducible subluxation of the hip: prognostic factors related to hip remodeling. J Bone Joint Surg 2009;91(10):1383–7.
14. Kamegaya M, Saisu T, Takazawa M, et al. Arthrographic indicators for decision making about femoral varus osteotomy in Legg-Calvé-Perthes disease. J Child Orthop 2008;2(4):261–7.
15. Napiontek M, Pietrzak S. Double osteotomy in the surgical treatment of Perthes disease: dega's transiliac osteotomy and subtrochanteric osteotomy. Ortop Traumatol Rehabil 2004;6(6):728–32.
16. Javid M, Wedge JH. Radiographic results of combined Salter innominate and femoral osteotomy in Legg-Calve-Perthes disease in older children. J Child Orthop 2009;3(3):229–34.

17. Vukasinovic Z, Spasovski D, Vucetic C, et al. Triple pelvic osteotomy in the treatment of Legg-Calvé-Perthes disease. Int Orthop (SICOT) 2009;33(5): 1377–83.

18. Conroy E, Sheehan E, O'Connor P, et al. Triple pelvic osteotomy in Legg-Calvé-Perthes disease using a single anterolateral incision: a 4-year review. J Pediatr Orthop B 2010;19(4):323–6.

19. Kruse RW, Guille JT, Bowen JR. Shelf arthroplasty in patients who have Legg-Calve-Perthes disease. J Bone Joint Surg Am 1991;73(9):1338–47.

20. Domzalski ME, Glutting J, Bowen JR, et al. Lateral acetabular growth stimulation following a labral support procedure in Legg-Calvé-Perthes disease. J Bone Joint Surg 2006;88(7):1450–66.

21. Robinson HJ, Sigmond MB, O'Connor S, et al. Innominate osteotomy in Perthes' disease. J Pediatr Orthop 1988;8(4):426–35.

22. Bennett JT, Mazurek RT, Cash JD. Chiari's osteotomy in the treatment of Perthes disease. J Bone Joint Surg 1991;73(2):225–8.

23. Joseph B, Mulpuri K, Vargheses G. Perthes' disease in the adolescent. J Bone Joint Surg 2001;83(5):715–20.

24. Bankes MJ, Catterall A, Hashemi-Nejad A. Valgus extension osteotomy for "hinge abduction" in Perthes' disease: results at maturity and factors influencing the radiological outcome. J Bone Joint Surg 2000;82B(4): 548–54.

25. Myers GJC, Mathur K, O'Hara J. Valgus osteotomy. A solution for late presentation of hinge abduction in Legg-Calvé-Perthes disease. J Pediatr Orthop 2008;28(2):169–72.

26. Freeman RT, Wainwright AM, Theologis TN, et al. The outcome of patients with hinge abduction in severe Perthes disease treated by shelf acetabuloplasty. J Pediatr Orthop 2008;28(6):619–25.

27. Canadell J, Gonzales F, Barrios RH, et al. Arthrodiatasis for stiff hips in young patients. Int Orthop 1993; 17(4):254–8.

28. Kocaoglu M, Kilicoglu OI, Goksan SB. Ilizarov fixator for treatment of Legg-Calvé-Perthes disease. J Pediatr Orthop B 1999;8(4):276–81.

29. Kukukkaya M, Kabukcuoglu Y, Ozturk I, et al. Avascular necrosis of the femoral head in childhood. the results of treatment with articulated distraction method. J Pediatr Orthop 2000;20(6):722–8.

30. Segev E, Ezra E, Wientroub S, et al. Treatment of severe late onset Perthes' disease with soft tissue release and articulated hip distraction: early results. J Pediatr Orthop B 2004;13(3):158–65.

31. Maxwell SL, Lappin KJ, Kealey WD, et al. Arthrodiatasis in Perthes' disease. Preliminary results. J Bone Joint Surg Br 2004;86(2):244–50.

32. Shin SJ, Kwak HS, Cho TJ, et al. Application of Ganz surgical hip dislocation in pediatric hip disease. Clin Orthop Surg 2009;1(3):132–7.

Valgus Osteotomy for Hinge Abduction

Antoine de Gheldere, MD[a], Deborah M. Eastwood, FRCS[b],*

KEYWORDS

- Valgus osteotomy • Legg-Calvé-Perthes disease
- Hinge abduction

Hinge abduction in Perthes disease was first described in the 1980s.[1,2] The investigators described an abnormal movement of the hip during abduction associated with significant restriction of movement and pain. The abnormal movement cannot be detected clinically (although the restriction can). Arthrography under general anesthesia demonstrates an increase in medial pooling with abduction, suggesting an impingement of the lateral (or anterolateral) part of the enlarged and deformed cartilaginous femoral head on the lateral portion of the acetabulum. Some investigators have tried to quantify the widening of the medial joint space on plain films,[3] whilst others have used different imaging techniques to describe the same phenomenon.[4,5] Nevertheless, failure of the lateral (or anterolateral) part of the femoral head to roll into the acetabulum changes the biomechanics of the hip joint such that it then works like a hinge in abduction. Hinge abduction is accepted as a poor prognostic factor,[1,2,6,7] and rapid progression to secondary osteoarthritis can be expected.[8,9]

AIM OF TREATMENT

In cases of hinge abduction, the goal of the valgus osteotomy is not to reconstruct an anatomic hip joint, but to improve joint biomechanics by restoring the rolling motion of the femoral head into the acetabulum and joint congruity in the weight-bearing position. It does so by effectively moving the area of femoral head deformity away from the acetabulum and its labrum, hence off-loading it and making the spherical medial part of the femoral head load bearing. The procedure will never restore a full range of motion to the hip joint but it will reorient the arc of congruent joint movement, allowing abduction without hinging within the physiologic range. The valgus osteotomy also has the capacity to lengthen the leg and to lower the greater trochanter, thus improving the articulotrochanteric distance. This process improves the abductor lever arm and hence its efficiency. Thus, a valgus proximal femoral osteotomy relieves groin pain, and provides a better and more efficient functional range of motion for the patient. If designed appropriately, the procedure can also reduce the leg length difference, and all of these factors improve gait pattern and the long-term remodeling of the hip joint.

TIMING OF SURGERY

The timing of the surgery is crucial. By opting for the valgus osteotomy, the surgeon accepts that he or she is "salvaging" a poor mechanical situation and that a containment procedure would be ineffective. It is essential to the success of this procedure that the quality of the bone in the superomedial region of the femoral head is good enough to withstand the forces associated with weight bearing once it is redirected into a weight-bearing position.

The femoral head deformity associated with hinge abduction occurs almost exclusively in cases of major involvement of the femoral epiphysis.[10] The Perthes disease should be in

No funding support.

No financial disclosures/conflicts of interest.

[a] Department of Orthopaedics, The Great North Children's Hospital, Queen Victoria Road, Newcastle upon Tyne NE1 4LP, UK

[b] The Catterall Unit, The Royal National Orthopaedic Hospital, Brockley Hill, Stanmore, Middlesex HA7 4LP, UK

* Corresponding author.

E-mail address: d.m.eastwood@btinternet.com

Orthop Clin N Am 42 (2011) 349–354

doi:10.1016/j.ocl.2011.04.005

the healing stage before this osteotomy is considered. This situation can be judged on plain radiographs if there is significant ossification in the healing phase, but in the late fragmentation phase a magnetic resonance imaging (MRI) scan with intravenous gadolinium injection gives a better assessment of the revascularization of the femoral head.[11] As a valgus osteotomy is a salvage procedure, there is little to be gained from performing the surgery too early.

PREOPERATIVE ASSESSMENT
Symptoms

The patient often presents with a relatively sudden deterioration in range of movement associated with significant pain, due to the abnormal joint biomechanics rather than the Perthes process itself.

Signs

The limp is confirmed on walking and a Trendelenburg sign is obvious. Measurement of the leg length discrepancy with blocks estimates the shortening of the involved hip and highlights the pelvic obliquity: care must be taken if there is a fixed adduction deformity. The reduction of hip movement, especially abduction, may be due to pain, muscle spasm, or femoral head deformity: limited abduction does not necessarily indicate

hinge abduction. Further investigation is required to confirm the diagnosis.

Investigation

Despite the comments of some investigators,[4] hinge abduction is a dynamic process. Thus preoperatively, it needs dynamic assessment: the static investigations of MRI and computed tomography scanning have a limited role. The most valuable investigation is a clinical examination combined with arthrography, performed under general anesthesia when all muscle spasm due to pain is absent. Leg length difference and fixed deformities must be documented: each may exacerbate the problems of hinge abduction and influence the choice of treatment. Following introduction of 2 to 3 mL of contrast material (Omnipaque 240/300; GE Healthcare, Amersham, UK) into the joint, an assessment of overall size and shape of the femoral head is made. Then the quality of femoroacetabular movement is assessed: as the leg is abducted, the sign of hinge abduction is noted with medial pooling of the dye and deformation of the lateral labrum (**Fig. 1**). Such unstable movement may also be demonstrated with internal/external rotation of the femoral head in extension. The dynamic arthrogram also allows identification of the "position of best fit," around which there is a cone of movement where there is congruity between the femoral head and the acetabulum. This position

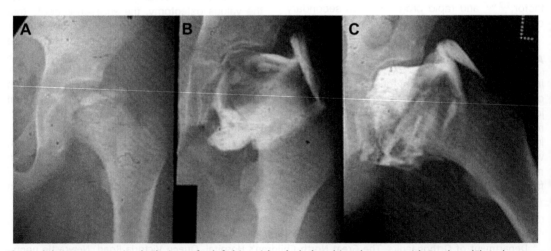

Fig. 1. (*A*) Anteroposterior (AP) view of a left hip with whole head involvement with Perthes. (*B*) Arthrogram with the femur in slight adduction, demonstrating a flattening of the cartilaginous femoral head and a well-shaped cartilaginous acetabular labrum. (*C*) The arthrogram demonstrates hinge abduction with medial pooling and deformation of the cartilaginous labrum as the femur has moved into abduction. (*From* Quain S, Catterall A. Hinge abduction of the hip. Diagnosis and treatment. J Bone Joint Surg Br 1986;68:62; with permission.)

is usually in 15°–25° of adduction with sometimes a few degrees of flexion.

OPERATIVE TECHNIQUE

The procedure is performed under general anesthesia. A femoral block or a caudal block can be administered for postoperative analgesia. The child is supine on a radiolucent table, providing access for the image intensifier. A radiolucent "sandbag" may be placed under the ipsilateral buttock to lift the greater trochanter.

A lateral incision is made from the tip of the greater trochanter distally along the longitudinal axis of the femur. The fascia lata is split in the line of the incision. The femoral insertion of gluteus maximus is identified posteriorly. At this level, a Hohmann retractor elevates the vastus lateralis anteriorly to expose the periosteum. This is split longitudinally, and proximally the cut is directed anteriorly to release the insertion of the vastus lateralis tendon and expose the distal greater trochanter. The periosteum is elevated with a Cobb spatula. Hohmann retractors are then used to expose the intertrochanteric and subtrochanteric femur.

A variety of implants are available for fixation of proximal femoral osteotomies in children and adolescents. The operative technique differs slightly depending on the device used (**Figs. 2** and **3**). The object of surgery is to place the hip in the "position of best fit" as defined on the preoperative arthrogram. If the osteotomy was designed to correct a fixed flexion deformity and/or the position of best fit was in flexion, an extension osteotomy is created and the laterally based bone wedge created by the osteotomy cuts will be wider posteriorly than anteriorly. Lateralization of the distal shaft is recommended to effectively lengthen the femoral neck, preserve the anatomic axis, and improve the mechanics of the hip joint. An oblique osteotomy will also lead to an improvement in leg length.

POSTOPERATIVE CARE

Analgesic medication is provided by either a patient-controlled or nurse-controlled pump. There is no need for a spica cast. The authors' preferred postoperative regime is to support the weight of the leg by slings and springs passing around the thigh and calf (**Fig. 4**). Early passive and active mobilization commences with extension of the hip and knee, followed by joint movement in all other directions. Once the child is comfortable, with good muscle control (particularly hamstrings and quadriceps) and a good range of movement at the hip joint, mobilization by toe-touch weight bearing with crutches is allowed. Progression from partial to full weight bearing is permitted at 6 weeks as the osteotomy unites.

DISCUSSION

The exact definition of hinge abduction remains controversial.[1–6] The authors believe that the combination of limited abduction (on clinical examination) with a deformed femoral head (as seen on plain radiographs) is not enough to confirm the diagnosis of hinge abduction. Assessment with a dynamic arthrogram is essential to demonstrate the unstable movement that occurs as the deformed and overgrown femoral head hinges on the unstable lateral segment of the unossified acetabulum (hinge abduction), and to determine the position of best fit in order to plan the corrective osteotomy. Hinge abduction, which occurs within a physiologic weight-bearing range and which is secondary to significant femoral head deformity, will only benefit from a valgus osteotomy in terms of joint congruency and hip biomechanics. In the original series of Quain and Catterall,[8] 20 of 23 patients had such limitation of abduction that to examination they were in fixed adduction: the valgus (extension) femoral osteotomy was promoted as a solution for this select patient group. In that article,[8] avascular necrosis due to other causes was also treated by this technique, and others[12] have similarly extended the indications for this procedure. However, the authors believe that in some cases the concept of a valgus osteotomy designed to move the femoral head deformity away from the acetabular edge has become confused with the principle of a valgus osteotomy that simply improves the articulotrochanteric distance, leg length, and hip mechanics without the need to address the problem of true hinge abduction. The term hinge abduction was originally described in relation to significant restriction of movement: it is now used more loosely and is applied to any abnormal movement even if it occurs outside the physiologic weight-bearing range. Assuming that leg lengths are within 1 to 2 cm of each other, hinge abduction is not significant if it only occurs with greater than 20° to 30° of abduction.

The femoral valgus osteotomy for hinge abduction aims to salvage a mechanically poor situation: if it is performed too early whilst the superomedial femoral head is in the fragmentation phase, there is a risk of recurrent femoral head deformity as this segment moves into the weight-bearing area.[10] If the procedure is performed later, after the femoral head has healed but failed to remodel

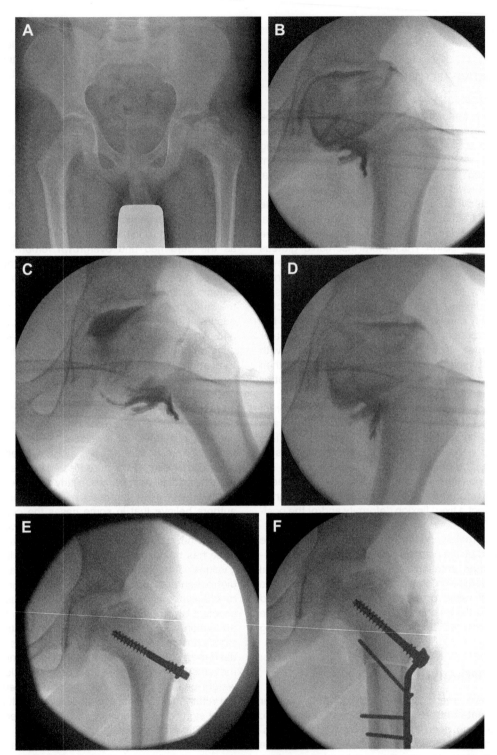

Fig. 2. (*A*) AP radiograph of a left hip with whole head involvement with Perthes. (*B*) Arthrogram with the left leg in neutral. The joint is incongruous and the acetabular labrum is being compressed. (*C*) Arthrogram with the left leg in abduction. There is gross medial dye pooling, and the cartilaginous acetabular labrum is displaced and deformed. (*D*) Arthrogram with the left leg in adduction. This is the position of "best fit" where there is minimal pooling and the labral shape is improved. (*E*) Coventry Screw (Ortho Solutions, Essex, UK) in position in the left femoral neck with the leg in neutral prior to osteotomy. (*F*) Following a 15° correction, the valgus osteotomy has been stabilized with a Coventry Screw and Plate system (Ortho Solutions) using an oblique screw across the osteotomy for additional rotational stability.

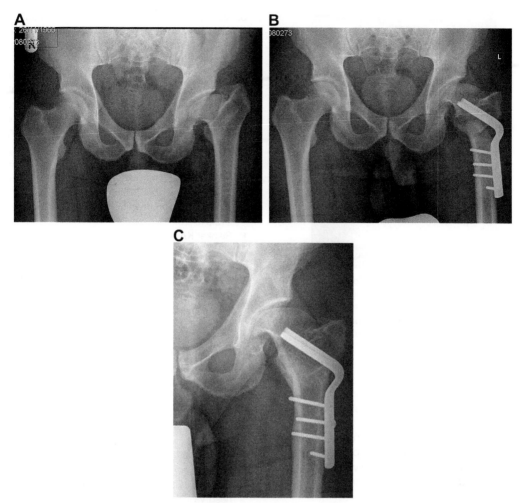

Fig. 3. (*A*) AP pelvic radiograph of a 40-year-old man with symptoms secondary to hinge abduction following Perthes disease as a child. (*B*) AP pelvic radiograph 3 weeks following a 30° valgus osteotomy stabilized with an AO blade plate (Synthes, Paoli, PA, USA). The articulotrochanteric distance has been improved, the shaft lateralized, and the leg effectively lengthened. (*C*) AP radiograph of the left hip 12 months following a valgus osteotomy. The osteotomy has united and the patient is asymptomatic.

well, recurrent deformity is less likely but there may be less opportunity for acetabular remodeling to improve joint congruity. A procedure performed when the femoral head has healed but while the triradiate cartilage is still open is more likely to be associated with acetabular remodeling and improved joint congruity.[10] Lateral acetabular growth may improve significantly and rapidly once hinging is abolished.[7]

Preoperative graphic planning makes the technique simple to use and, if necessary, correction in 3 planes is possible. The plate and screw system can be used for children; however, the authors prefer a blade plate system for adolescents.

The procedure provides reliable short-term relief of pain with an improvement in hip range of movement (particularly abduction).[7,8,12] Long-term results are also good following valgus osteotomy, valgus extension, or multidirectional correction.[7,10,12] Similar success has been reported in skeletally mature patients[12,13] and when the femoral head deformity is attributable to causes other than Perthes.[8,12]

Many patients with Perthes disease demonstrate a Shapiro type 4 pattern of abnormal growth[14] during their adolescent years, and thus an additional trochanteric epiphysiodesis or distal transfer, or a contralateral distal femoral/proximal tibial epiphysiodesis may be required. Leg lengths should be equal at skeletal maturity.

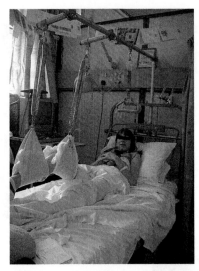

Fig. 4. Postoperative rehabilitation following a valgus osteotomy: the weight of the right leg is supported by the slings and springs, allowing ease of movement, and encouraging early active and passive hip range of movement and strengthening exercises.

SUMMARY

Proximal femoral valgus (extension) osteotomy is an effective procedure for the relief of the pain associated with hinge abduction. It improves the functional range of motion of the hip and thus the biomechanics. This salvage procedure can achieve many years of hip survival and will not compromise a future total hip arthroplasty.

ACKNOWLEDGMENTS

Both authors are indebted to Anthony Catterall: his wisdom, teaching, and support have been influential in helping us care for our patients and improve our understanding of pediatric orthopedics.

REFERENCES

1. Catterall A. Legg-Calvé-Perthes syndrome. Clin Orthop Relat Res 1981;158:41–52.
2. Grossbard GD. Hip pain during adolescence after Perthes' disease. J Bone Joint Surg Br 1981;63(4): 572–4.
3. Kruse RW, Guille JT, Bowen JR. Shelf arthroplasty in patients who have Legg-Calvé-Perthes disease. A study of long-term results. J Bone Joint Surg Am 1991;73:1338–47.
4. Kim HT, Wenger DR. Surgical correction of "functional retroversion" and "functional coxa vara" in late Legg-Calvé-Perthes disease and epiphyseal dysplasia: correction of deformity defined by new imaging modalities. J Pediatr Orthop 1997;17: 247–54.
5. Jaramillo D, Galen TA, Winalski CS, et al. Legg-Calvé-Perthes disease: MR imaging evaluation during manual positioning of the hip—comparison with conventional arthrography. Radiology 1999; 212:519–25.
6. Reinker KA. Early diagnosis and treatment of hinge abduction in Legg-Perthes disease. J Pediatr Orthop 1996;16:3–9.
7. Yoo WJ, Choi IH, Chung CY, et al. Valgus femoral osteotomy for hinge abduction in Perthes' disease. Decision-making and outcomes. J Bone Joint Surg Br 2004;86:726–30.
8. Quain S, Catterall A. Hinge abduction of the hip. Diagnosis and treatment. J Bone Joint Surg Br 1986;68:61–4.
9. Stulberg SD, Cooperman DR, Wallensten R. The natural history of Legg-Calvé-Perthes disease. J Bone Joint Surg Am 1981;63:1095–108.
10. Bankes MJ, Catterall A, Hashemi-Nejad A. Valgus extension osteotomy for hinge abduction in Perthes' disease. J Bone Joint Surg Br 2000;82: 548–54.
11. Lamer S, Dorgeret S, Khairouni A, et al. Femoral head vascularisation in Legg-Calvé-Perthes disease: comparison of dynamic gadolinium-enhanced subtraction MRI with bone scintigraphy. Pediatr Radiol 2002; 32:580–5.
12. Patil S, Sherlock D. Valgus osteotomy for hinge abduction in avascular necrosis. J Pediatr Orthop B 2006;15:262–6.
13. Myers GJ, Mathur K, O'Hara J. Valgus osteotomy: a solution for late presentation of hinge abduction in Legg-Calvé-Perthes disease. J Pediatr Orthop 2008;281:69–72.
14. Shapiro F. Developmental patterns in lower-extremity length discrepancies. J Bone Joint Surg Am 1982; 64:639–51.

Shelf and/or Reduction and Containment Surgery

Kent A. Reinker, MD*

KEYWORDS

- Legg-Calvé-Perthes disease • Hinge abduction
- Shelf procedure • Iliac osteotomy
- Femoral osteotomy • Hip

Hinge abduction was first described by Catterall and by Grossbard in 1981.[1,2] Since then, many authors have further elucidated the concept.[3–17] It is now known that

- Hinge abduction is present in 5% to 20% of hips with Legg-Perthes disease.
- Hinge abduction can occur early in fragmentation phase, before the hip can be accurately classified by either the Herring lateral pillar[18,19] or the Catterall[20] methods.
- The earliest clinical signs are loss of abduction and internal rotation of the hip.
- As early hinge abduction occurs due to impingement on unossified cartilage, standard anteroposterior and frog lateral radiographs are unable to visualize it.
- Hips with unrelieved hinge abduction have a very poor prognosis.

The best means of diagnosing hinge abduction is controversial. Most authors continue to use arthrography, as originally described, as the definitive radiographic test.[1,2,5,7,17,21] Nakamura, citing the subjectivity of classical arthrographic diagnosis, devised an acetabular index, in which the medial cartilage space is divided by the acetabular width. Increase of this index with abduction is then taken as indicative of hinge abduction.[7] This index corrects for magnification errors that might be present when using the image intensifier.

Reinker, seeking a diagnostic criterion available in the outpatient clinic, found that failure of the lateral pillar to pass under the acetabular edge with abduction of the internally rotated and extended hip was indicative of hinge abduction.[11] This criterion is somewhat more stringent than the arthrographic criteria, as some hips that meet this test do not demonstrate hinge abduction on arthrography. The question is whether the general anesthesia used for the arthrogram masks hinge abduction that is present when the patient is awake. Should these patients then be treated as though they had hinge abduction or not? This question is unanswered at present. The author and colleagues have taken the view that these patients do have hinge abduction, but that it is reversible. They have treated them with abduction casts for 6 to 8 weeks. If the lateral pillar remains under the edge of the acetabulum, the author and colleagues treat them as they do patients without hinge abduction. If, however, patients are unable to maintain the hip in the reduced position, the author and colleagues treat them as though they have persistent hinge abduction.

TREATMENT

The treatment of patients with hinge abduction is controversial, but basically involves one of 4 types:

1. Acetabular augmentation, either by Chiari osteotomy or by shelf arthroplasty; in either case, the goal is to remove the impingement on the acetabular edge by extending the effective edge of the acetabulum over the extruded portion of the femoral head

The author received no funding support for this article and has no financial disclosures relevant to this article.
Department of Orthopaedics, University of Texas Health Sciences Center, MC 7774, 7703 Floyd Curl Drive, San Antonio, TX 78229, USA
* 13637 Bluff Circle, San Antonio, TX 78216.
E-mail address: kreinker@mac.com

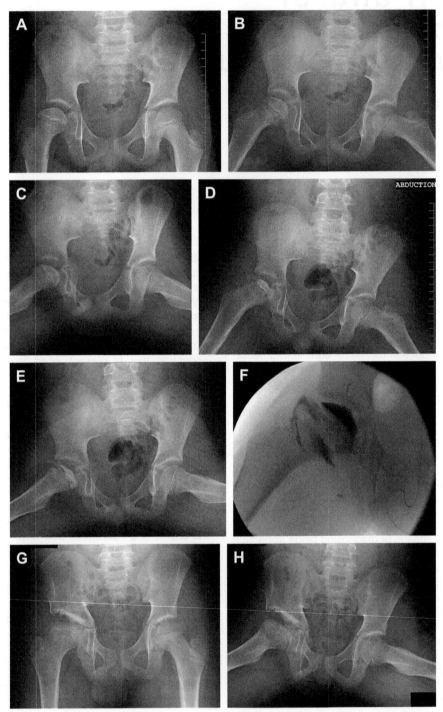

Fig. 1. (*A–C*) Anteroposterior, Abduction, and lateral radiographs of an 8-year-old boy with Perthes disease in early fragmentation phase. Abduction is limited to 15°. Failure of the capital epiphysis to slide under the acetabulum is indicative of hinge abduction. (*D, E*) Six months later, the epiphysis is flattened, and hinge abduction is now obvious on the abduction view. (*F*) Arthrogram confirms hinge abduction. (*G, H*) Three years after Chiari osteotomy, the femoral head is ovoid but improving. Range of motion now matches the opposite side.

2. Valgus femoral osteotomy, such that the impingement does not occur until the femur is widely abducted
3. Reshaping of the femoral head or neck, with impinging structures being removed
4. Capsulotomy to obtain reduction, followed by additional treatment as necessary.

Chiari osteotomy is a well-established procedure in the treatment of Legg-Perthes disease, with good results being reported by many authors (Fig. 1).[11,22-37] Cahuzac performed 17 Chiari osteotomies in Legg-Perthes patients and reported 12 having regular femoral heads postoperatively, 4 irregular, and 1 very irregular.[25] Fourteen patients were pain free at maturity. Bennett reported on 17 patients who had Chiari osteotomy with "painful, incongruent, subluxed hips." At review, significant improvements of centre-edge angle and percent coverage were documented. No patients reported pain with normal activity. Using the Mitchell classification system,[38] 12 were rated fair, and 1 poor. Reddy, in a series largely composed of patients with demonstrated hinge abduction, documented significant improvement of femoral head sphericity after Chiari osteotomy at mean age of 8.5 years. At maturity, 68% of patients were in Stulberg class 2, 18% Stulberg 3, and 14% Stulberg 4.[36,39] Abduction and internal rotation improved in 72% of cases. Pain was relieved completely in 73% of patients, with 27% of patients having occasional painful episodes.

The value of shelf arthroplasty has also been well documented in the treatment of Legg-Perthes disease.[5,40-49] Some have considered that shelf arthroplasty is contraindicated in the presence of hinge abduction.[40-42,49] Kruse, however, reported good long-term results in patients with hinge abduction treated at a mean age of 8 years with preoperative traction, adducter tenotomy, and shelf arthroplasty.[5] After mean 19 years of follow-up, 15 of the 20 hips were able to have Stulberg grading. Two hips were Stulberg class 2, seven class 3, five class 4 and one class 5. He was able to eliminate hinge abduction in 11 of 14 patients.

Freeman, in a study of shelf arthroplasty limited to patients having hinge abduction, documented excellent results, with 1 patient rated as Stulberg 1, 13 as Stulberg 2, 10 as Stulberg 3, two as Stulberg 4 and one as Stulberg 5. They documented a "striking" improvement of pain almost immediately postoperatively, with 24 of 28 patients being pain-free at final follow-up.

The rationale for capsulotomy is to decrease force at the acetabular edge by allowing greater abduction before the medial capsule becomes tight and creates a nutcracker effect on the femoral head. Capsular release has the potential, however, for allowing an increase in the degree of subluxation when the hip is adducted. The author and colleagues therefore view this as a possibly helpful adjunct to other techniques. Very little information is available about the results of capsular release.[50]

DISCUSSION

The best treatment for patients with hinge abduction continues to be controversial; however, much has been learned during the past decade, and good results have now been reported even with patients with severe deformity. Treatment of patients without hinge abduction is discussed in other articles.[51-55] For the patient in whom hinge abduction is suspected, the author and colleagues obtain an abduction/internal rotation/extension radiograph. If this shows hinge abduction, the author and colleagues do arthrography. If the arthrogram shows reversible or absent hinge abduction, or if the extruded fragment can be covered adequately by a shelf, a shelf arthroplasty is performed. If a reasonable sized shelf would not adequately cover the femoral head, the author and colleagues perform Chiari osteotomy. The author and colleagues reserve valgus osteotomy for late patients with hinge abduction who are well into the regenerative phase of disease, as they feel that the literature shows better results from augmentation arthroplasty than for valgus osteotomy in patients treated early in the course. The author and colleagues continue to view cheilectomy as a last resort, to be used when range of motion is so poor that femoral osteotomy is unlikely to lead to an adequate result.

REFERENCES

1. Catterall A. Legg-Calve-Perthes syndrome. Clin Orthop Relat Res 1981;(158):41–52.
2. Grossbard GD. Hip pain during adolescence after Perthes' disease. J Bone Joint Surg Br 1981;63:572.
3. Arkader A, Sankar WN, Amorim RM. Conservative versus surgical treatment of late-onset Legg-Calve-Perthes disease: a radiographic comparison at skeletal maturity. J Child Orthop 2009;3:21.
4. Harrison MH. A preliminary account of the management of the painful hip originating from Perthes' disease. Clin Orthop Relat Res 1986;(209):57–64.
5. Kruse RW, Guille JT, Bowen JR. Shelf arthroplasty in patients who have Legg-Calve-Perthes disease. A study of long-term results. J Bone Joint Surg Am 1991;73:1338.
6. Kuwajima SS, Crawford AH, Ishida A, et al. Comparison between Salter's innominate osteotomy and

augmented acetabuloplasty in the treatment of patients with severe Legg-Calve-Perthes disease. Analysis of 90 hips with special reference to roentgenographic sphericity and coverage of the femoral head. J Pediatr Orthop B 2002;11:15.

7. Nakamura J, Kamegaya M, Saisu T, et al. Hip arthrography under general anesthesia to refine the definition of hinge abduction in Legg-Calve-Perthes disease. J Pediatr Orthop 2008;28:614.

8. Oh CW, Rodriguez A, Guille JT, et al. Labral support shelf arthroplasty for the early stages of severe Legg-Calve-Perthes disease. Am J Orthop (Belle Mead NJ) 2010;39:26–9.

9. Patil S, Sherlock D. Valgus osteotomy for hinge abduction in avascular noorosis. J Pediatr Orthop B 2006;15:262.

10. Quain S, Catterall A. Hinge abduction of the hip. Diagnosis and treatment. J Bone Joint Surg Br 1986;68:61.

11. Reinker KA. Early diagnosis and treatment of hinge abduction in Legg-Perthes disease. J Pediatr Orthop 1996;16:3.

12. Reinker KA, Larsen IJ. Patterns of progression in Legg-Perthes disease. J Pediatr Orthop 1983;3:455.

13. Rowe SM, Jung ST, Cheon SY, et al. Outcome of cheilectomy in Legg-Calve-Perthes disease: minimum 25-year follow-up of five patients. J Pediatr Orthop 2006;26:204.

14. Roy DR. Arthroscopy of the hip in children and adolescents. J Child Orthop 2009;3:89.

15. Shin SJ, Kwak HS, Cho TJ, et al. Application of ganz surgical hip dislocation approach in pediatric hip diseases. Clin Orthop Surg 2009;1:132.

16. Snow SW, Keret D, Scarangella S, et al. Anterior impingement of the femoral head: a late phenomenon of Legg-Calve-Perthes' disease. J Pediatr Orthop 1993;13:286.

17. Urlus M, Stoffelen D, Fabry G. Hinge abduction in avascular necrosis of the hip: diagnosis and treatment. J Pediatr Orthop B 1992;1:67.

18. Herring JA, Kim HT, Browne R. Legg-Calve-Perthes disease. Part I: classification of radiographs with use of the modified lateral pillar and Stulberg classifications. J Bone Joint Surg Am 2004;86:2103.

19. Herring JA, Kim HT, Browne R. Legg-Calve-Perthes disease. Part II: prospective multicenter study of the effect of treatment on outcome. J Bone Joint Surg Am 2004;86:2121.

20. Catterall A. Natural history, classification, and x-ray signs in Legg-Calve-Perthes disease. Acta Orthop Belg 1980;46:346.

21. Yoo WJ, Choi IH, Chung CY, et al. Valgus femoral osteotomy for hinge abduction in Perthes' disease. Decision-making and outcomes. J Bone Joint Surg Br 2004;86:726.

22. Bailey TE Jr, Hall JE. Chiari medial displacement osteotomy. J Pediatr Orthop 1985;5:635.

23. Bankes MJ, Catterall A, Hashemi-Nejad A. Valgus extension osteotomy for hinge abduction in Perthes' disease. Results at maturity and factors influencing the radiological outcome. J Bone Joint Surg Br 2000;82:548.

24. Bennett JT, Mazurek RT, Cash JD. Chiari's osteotomy in the treatment of Perthes' disease. J Bone Joint Surg Br 1991;73:225.

25. Cahuzac JP, Onimus M, Trottmann F, et al. Chiari pelvic osteotomy in Perthes disease. J Pediatr Orthop 1990;10:163.

26. Canario AT, Williams L, Wientroub S, et al. A controlled study of the results of femoral osteotomy in severe Perthes' disease. J Bone Joint Surg Br 1980;62:438.

27. Castaneda P, Haynes R, Mijares J, et al. Varus-producing osteotomy for patients with lateral pillar type B and C Legg-Calve-Perthes disease followed to skeletal maturity. J Child Orthop 2008;2:373.

28. Catterall A. Adolescent hip pain after Perthes' disease. Clin Orthop Relat Res 1986;(209):65–9.

29. Chairi K, Endler M, Hackel H. Treatment of coxa magna in Perthes disease by pelvic osteotomy. Arch Orthop Trauma Surg 1978;91:183.

30. Graham S, Westin GW, Dawson E, et al. The Chiari osteotomy. A review of 58 cases. Clin Orthop Relat Res 1986;(208):249–58.

31. Kerschbaumer F, Bauer R. The Chiari pelvic osteotomy—indications and results. Arch Orthop Trauma Surg 1979;95:51.

32. Kim HT, Wenger DR. Functional retroversion of the femoral head in Legg-Calve-Perthes disease and epiphyseal dysplasia: analysis of head–neck deformity and its effect on limb position using three-dimensional computed tomography. J Pediatr Orthop 1997;17:240.

33. Kim HT, Wenger DR. Surgical correction of functional retroversion and functional coxa vara in late Legg-Calve-Perthes disease and epiphyseal dysplasia: correction of deformity defined by new imaging modalities. J Pediatr Orthop 1997;17:247.

34. Koyama K, Higuchi F, Inoue A. Modified Chiari osteotomy for arthrosis after Perthes' disease. 14 hips followed for 2–12 years. Acta Orthop Scand 1998;69:129.

35. Lack W, Feldner-Busztin H, Ritschl P, et al. The results of surgical treatment for Perthes' disease. J Pediatr Orthop 1989;9:197.

36. Reddy RR, Morin C. Chiari osteotomy in Legg-Calve-Perthes disease. J Pediatr Orthop B 2005;14:1.

37. Vukasinovic Z, Vucetic C, Spasovski D, et al. Legg-Calve-Perthes disease-diagnostics and contemporary treatment. SrpArhCelok Lek 2008;136:430 [in Serbian].

38. Mitchell GP. Chiari medial displacement osteotomy. Clin Orthop Relat Res 1974;(98):146–50.

39. Stulberg SD, Cooperman DR, Wallensten R. The natural history of Legg-Calve-Perthes disease. J Bone Joint Surg Am 1981;63:1095.

40. Bursal A, Erkula G. Lateral shelf acetabuloplasty in the treatment of Legg-Calve-Perthes disease. J Pediatr Orthop B 2004;13:150.

41. Daly K, Bruce C, Catterall A. Lateral shelf acetabuloplasty in Perthes' disease. A review of the end of growth. J Bone Joint Surg Br 1999;81:380.

42. Domzalski ME, Glutting J, Bowen JR, et al. Lateral acetabular growth stimulation following a labral support procedure in Legg-Calve-Perthes disease. J Bone Joint Surg Am 2006;88:1458.

43. Eijer H, Podeszwa DA, Ganz R, et al. Evaluation and treatment of young adults with femoro-acetabular impingement secondary to Perthes' disease. Hip Int 2006;16:273.

44. Freeman RT, Wainwright AM, Theologis TN, et al. The outcome of patients with hinge abduction in severe Perthes disease treated by shelf acetabuloplasty. J Pediatr Orthop 2008;28:619.

45. Garceau G. Surgical treatment of coxa plana. J Bone Joint Surg Br 1964;46:779.

46. Jacobs R, Moens P, Fabry G. Lateral shelf acetabuloplasty in the early stage of Legg-Calve-Perthes disease with special emphasis on the remaining growth of the acetabulum: a preliminary report. J Pediatr Orthop B 2004;13:21.

47. Pecquery R, Laville JM, Salmeron F. Legg-Calve-Perthes disease treatment by augmentation acetabuloplasty. Orthop Traumatol Surg Res 2010; 96:166.

48. Van Der Geest IC, Kooijman MA, Spruit M, et al. Shelf acetabuloplasty for Perthes' disease: 12-year follow-up. Acta Orthop Belg 2001;67:126.

49. Yoo WJ, Choi IH, Cho TJ, et al. Shelf acetabuloplasty for children with Perthes' disease and reducible subluxation of the hip: prognostic factors related to hip remodelling. J Bone Joint Surg Br 2009;91:1383.

50. Mehlman CT, Parker KC, Roy DR, et al. Hinge abduction and joint stiffness in Perthes disease: effectiveness of medial soft tissue release and Petrieasting followed by femoral head containment (poster# 39). In: 67th AAOS annual meeting proceedings. Orlando (FL): American Academy of Orthopedics Surgeons; 2000. p. 451.

51. Lloyd-Roberts GC, Catterall A, Salamon PB. A controlled study of the indications for and the results of femoral osteotomy in Perthes' disease. J Bone Joint Surg Br 1976;58:31.

52. McKay DW. Cheilectomy of the hip. Orthop Clin North Am 1980;11:141.

53. de Sanctis N, Rega AN, Rondinella F. Prognostic evaluation of Legg-Calve-Perthes disease by MRI. Part I: the role of physeal involvement. J Pediatr Orthop 2000;20:455.

54. de Sanctis N, Rondinella F. Prognostic evaluation of Legg-Calve-Perthes disease by MRI. Part II: pathomorphogenesis and new classification. J Pediatr Orthop 2000;20:463.

55. Javid M, Wedge JH. Radiographic results of combined Salter innominate and femoral osteotomy in Legg-Calve-Perthes disease in older children. J Child Orthop 2009;3:229.

Articulated Distraction

Gamal Ahmed Hosny, MD

KEYWORDS

• Hip • Distraction • Perthes • Arthrodiatasis

Articulated distraction or arthrodiatasis is a new method of treatment of Legg-Calvé-Perthes disease (LCPD). The term arthrodiatasis is derived from the Greek words arthro (joint), dia (through), and taxis (to stretch out).[1] The method has been used to treat a variety of hip conditions, such as avascular necrosis, osteoarthritis, chondrolysis, neglected hip dislocation, unstable capital femoral epiphysis, and the adolescent arthritic hip.[2–5]

RATIONALE

The aim of treatment of LCPD is to prevent the residual hip deformity, which can lead to early degenerative arthritis.[6] During the stage of revascularization, the bone of the femoral head is biologically weak. When this weak bone is subjected to weight-bearing stresses across the edge of the acetabulum, the femoral head can become irreversibly deformed. Even when the hip is not bearing weight, muscular contraction can generate forces across the joint that may exceed the body weight; these forces can cause the femoral head to deform. Joint distraction attempts to neutralize muscular and weight-bearing forces on the femoral epiphysis, induce neovascularization, and prevent femoral head deformation.

One advantage of distraction is that it does not change the anatomy of the proximal femur. Besides, it can be employed even when the hip is very stiff, when other methods of surgical containment are contraindicated.[7]

METHODS

Articulated hip distraction can be applied with either a monolateral fixator or a circular external fixator. If fixed adduction or flexion deformities are present, tenotomies of the adductors and the psoas tendons are first performed.

Whatever the type of external fixator, it should be aligned such that its rotating axis is in line with the flexion–extension axis of the hip joint.[8] This step is crucial. If alignment of the center of rotation is not accurate, limitation of movement and even painful loosening of the pins may occur.[9] A guidewire is inserted from the lateral side through the center of rotation of the hip joint under image-intensifier control while the lower limb is kept in 15° abduction, neutral rotation, and 0° flexion. This position is used so that the guidewire is perpendicular to the femoral shaft. The hinge of the monolateral articulated distraction device is aligned with this guidewire (**Fig. 1**). Two half pins (5 or 6 mm) are inserted in the supra-acetabular area using the image intensifier for avoiding too-deep penetration. The author prefers the use of hydroxyapatite-coated pins. Another 2 or 3 pins are applied to the shaft of the femur in the midsagittal plane. The guide pin is removed and the range of motion of the hip is checked. A circular external fixator can be applied with the same principles as the monolateral hinged fixator. Schanz pins are introduced in a convergent manner into the iliac crest,[10,11] the supra-acetabular area, or both, and fixed to a pelvic arch. Another arch or a complete ring is applied to the femur by wires or pins. The connection between the two parts is built using rods and hinges, ensuring that the level of the hinge is at the center of hip rotation as previously described. In cases with flexion hip deformity, an extension rod can be applied for a temporary period to correct the deformity and restrict all movements.

The author has nothing to disclose.
Department of Orthopaedics, Benha Faculty of Medicine, Benha University, 53 Misr Helwan Street, Maadi, Cairo, Egypt
E-mail address: gamalahosny@yahoo.com

Orthop Clin N Am 42 (2011) 361–364
doi:10.1016/j.ocl.2011.04.010

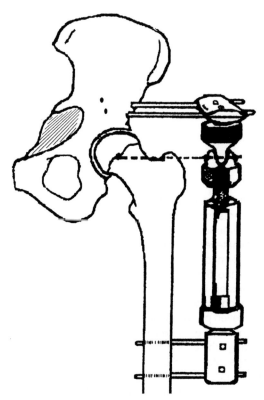

Fig. 1. Diagram showing that the hinge of the fixator has to be built on the center of the hip rotation. (*From* Canadell J, Gonzales F, Barrios RH, et al. Arthrodiastasis for stiff hips in young children. Int Orthop 1993;17:254–8; with permission.)

POSTOPERATIVE PROTOCOL

Patients are allowed to walk with partial weight bearing with crutches on the second day after the operation. A day later, distraction is started at a rate of 1 mm/d. Distraction is continued until the Shenton line is overcorrected by 5 to 10 mm (**Fig. 2**). Physiotherapy is performed daily to maintain hip flexion and extension. The end point of distraction is when adequate ossification of the lateral pillar is seen because no further collapse of the epiphysis is expected beyond this stage of the disease. This result would normally take 4 or 5 months in the fixator. After fixator removal, the child has daily hydrotherapy and physiotherapy with passive continuous and active assisted movements. Non–weight-bearing activity is recommended for 2 months.[12,13]

COMPLICATIONS

1. Pin-track infection is the most frequent complication. Usually, it responds to frequent dressing and oral or parenteral antibiotics. However,

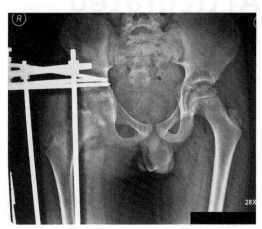

Fig. 2. Distraction of the right hip with overcorrection of the Shenton line.

premature removal of the fixator has been reported because of severe pin-track infection. There is a remote possibility of infection in cases where hip arthroplasty would be required in the future.
2. Pin breakage has been reported in obese patients.[7]
3. Mechanical failure of the fixator during distraction has been reported.[13,14] The surgeon must be aware of mechanical failure as a potential cause for lack of anticipated joint distraction during arthrodiatasis.
4. Subluxation after fixator removal had been reported in a few cases.[10,15] However, the coverage of the femoral head improved with longer follow-up.
5. Chondrodiatasis of the growth plate developed in 1 case with resultant femoral neck lengthening instead of arthrodiatasis. The accumulating tension during distraction was conveyed to the femoral epiphysis instead of the hip joint, probably because of marked intraarticular adhesions.[15]

Psychological intolerance that required fixator removal has not been reported.[11]

DISCUSSION

Only a few reports of arthrodiatasis in LCPD have appeared in the literature and not many centers advocate this form of treatment.[16]

A review of the published results describing this method of treatment of LCPD[1,10,11,13,15,17,18] is summarized in **Table 1**. Most of these reports share the same limitations: small number of patients, absence of a control group, relatively short follow-up, and diversity of indications.

Table 1
Comparison of the 6 articles of hip arthrodiatasis in LCPD

	Kocaoglu et al,[19] 1999	Maxwell et al,[17] 2004	Aly & Amin[1] 2009	Kucukkaya et al,[11] 2000	Segev et al,[18] 2007	Hosny et al,[15] 2011
Number of cases	11	15	23	8	10	29
Age	5–10 y	7.1–12.5 y	5–8 y	6–10 y	>9 y	>8 y
Lat pillar classification	B4 C7	A1 B14	B9 C14	B&C	Out of 16 cases in 2004 B1 C15	B5 C24
Follow-up period	24–50 mo	15.8–56.6 mo	52–104 mo	13–69 mo	4.3–7.8 y	2.9–11.0 y
Complications	Pin-track infection in 7 cases Translocation of the ring on the iliac crest Self disassembly of the device Subluxation in 2 cases	Pin-track infection in most of the cases Fracture pin in 2 cases Stiffness of the hip in 2 cases	Pin-track infection in 1 case	Pin-track infection in most of the cases Restriction of the hip Joint movement in 1 case	Reported before Segev et al,[13] 2004 Pin-track infection in 13 cases (out of 16) Broken clamp	Pin-track infection in 22 cases Chondrodiatasis instead of arthrodiatasis in 1 case Hip subluxation in 1 case
Stulburg classification	II 3 III 7 IV 1	Not applied in this study	Not applied in this study	II 4 cases III 3 cases V 1 case	III 3 cases IV 7 cases	Classification for 21 cases only II 9 cases III 7 cases IV 4 cases V 1 case
Type of distraction	9 cases nonarticulated 2 cases articulated Soft-tissue release in some cases	Articulated	Articulated and Soft-tissue release	Articulated	Articulated and Soft-tissue release	Nonarticulated No soft-tissue release
Control group	None	Yes	Yes	None	None	None

Although Aly and Amin[1] used the technique in children aged younger than 8 years as the primary method of containment, most investigators have used this method more frequently as a salvage procedure in the older child, or in children who present with severe forms of the disease and marked limitation of hip motion. Arthrodiatasis has also been advocated as a preliminary step before surgical containment in late-onset cases with increasing pain and decreased range of motion.[7]

The reported outcomes have varied a great deal. When articulated distraction was applied to hips with minimal collapse, the short-term results revealed preservation of the epiphyseal height.[17] However, long-term results have not been as encouraging; Segev and colleagues[18] reported that 7 of 10 cases had Stulberg class IV hips at final follow-up and the remaining 3 hips were graded as Stulberg class III hips. One clear benefit of articulated hip distraction noted by most investigators is improvement of joint stiffness.[12,13,15]

REFERENCES

1. Aly TA, Amin OA. Arthrodiatasis for the treatment of Perthes' disease. Orthopedics 2009;32(11):817.
2. Aldegheri R, Trivella G, Saleh M. Articulated distraction of the hip. Conservative surgery for arthritis in young patients. Clin Orthop Relat Res 1994;(301):94–101.
3. Thacker MM, Feldman DS, Madan SS, et al. Hinged distraction of the adolescent arthritic hip. J Pediatr Orthop 2005;25(2):178–82.
4. Nagarajah K, Aslam N, McLardy Smith P, et al. Iliofemoral distraction and hip reconstruction for the sequelae of a septic dislocated hip with chronic femoral osteomyelitis. J Bone Joint Surg Br 2005;87(6):863–6.
5. Song HR, Myrboh V, Lee SH. Unstable slipped capital femoral epiphysis: reduction by gradual distraction with external fixator. A case report. J Pediatr Orthop B 2005;14(6):426–8.
6. Salter RB. Legg-Perthes disease: the scientific basis for the methods of treatment and their indications. Clin Orthop Relat Res 1980;(150):8–11.
7. Sudesh P, Bali K, Mootha AK, et al. Arthrodiastasis and surgical containment in severe late-onset Perthes disease: an analysis of 14 patients. Acta Orthop Belg 2010;76(3):329–34.
8. Ozger H, Eralp L, Atalar AC. Articulated distraction of the hip joint in the treatment of benign aggressive tumors located around the hip joint. Arch Orthop Trauma Surg 2003;123(8):399–403.
9. Gomez JA, Matsumoto H, Roye DP Jr, et al. Articulated hip distraction: a treatment option for femoral head avascular necrosis in adolescence. J Pediatr Orthop 2009;29(2):163–9.
10. Kocaoglu M, Kilicoglu OI, Goksan SB, et al. Ilizarov fixator for treatment of Legg-Calvé-Perthes disease. J Pediatr Orthop B 1999;8(4):276–81.
11. Kucukkaya M, Kabukcuoglu Y, Ozturk I, et al. Avascular necrosis of the femoral head in childhood: the results of treatment with articulated distraction method. J Pediatr Orthop 2000;20(6):722–8.
12. Cañadell J, Gonzales F, Barrios RH, et al. Arthrodiastasis for stiff hips in young patients. Int Orthop 1993;17(4):254–8.
13. Segev E, Ezra E, Wientroub S, et al. Treatment of severe late onset Perthes' disease with soft tissue release and articulated hip distraction: early results. J Pediatr Orthop B 2004;13(3):158–65.
14. Sabharwal S, Van Why D. Mechanical failure of external fixator during hip joint distraction for Perthes disease. J Orthop Sci 2007;12(4):385–9.
15. Hosny GA, El-Deeb K, Fadel M, et al. Arthrodiatasis of the hip. J Pediatr Orthop, in press.
16. Hefti F, Clarke NM. The management of Legg-Calvé-Perthes' disease: is there a consensus?: a study of clinical practice preferred by the members of the European Paediatric Orthopaedic Society. J Child Orthop 2007;1(1):19–25.
17. Maxwell SL, Lappin KJ, Kealey WD, et al. Arthrodiastasis in Perthes' disease. Preliminary results. J Bone Joint Surg Br 2004;86(2):244–50.
18. Segev E, Ezra E, Wientroub S, et al. Treatment of severe late-onset Perthes' disease with soft tissue release and articulated hip distraction: revisited at skeletal maturity. J Child Orthop 2007;1(4):229–35.
19. Kocaoglu M, Kilicoglu OI, Goksan SB, et al. Ilizarov fixator for treatment of Legg-Calvé-Perthes disease. J Pediatr Orthop B 1999;8(4):276–81.

Principles of Treating the Sequelae of Perthes Disease

Dennis R. Wenger, MD*, Harish S. Hosalkar, MD

KEYWORDS

- Extra-articular osteotomy • Perthes disease
- Residual hip joint deformity
- Femoral head neck recontouring

Despite early treatment efforts, many patients with Perthes disease are left with residual femoral head deformity that can be symptomatic with a residual limp and poor hip motion. Containment treatment to restore sphericity of the femoral head is inappropriate in such cases. Selecting treatment methods for symptomatic patients with Perthes disease with healed but deformed femoral heads has always been difficult (**Fig. 1**) but is now even more complex because of the new possibilities of femoral head–neck recontouring and femoral head reduction surgery. Occasionally, patients develop osteochondritis dissecans when there is little femoral head deformity. The primary objective of management is to establish the exact cause of pain and address that cause specifically. This article outlines an approach to these patients. An outline of possible choices is presented in **Box 1**.

CLASSIFICATION OF SEQUELAE

Although new methods for identifying the sequelae of Perthes are emerging in the era of "hip impingement," the traditional Stulberg classification of the sequelae of Legg-Calvé-Perthes disease remains the standard. Stulberg and colleagues[1] described a system of classification that predicts the risk for early osteoarthritis on the basis of hip joint shape and congruity. Early onset arthritis is uncommon when the femoral head is spherical (Stulberg I and II), but some of these patients may have impingement symptoms and labral tears that interfere with physical activities. Patients with late

Perthes disease with Stulberg class III, IV, and V classification may develop early onset arthritis, but there are no current guidelines for prophylactic treatment.

TREATMENT OF RESIDUAL DEFORMITY WITH EXTRAARTICULAR PROCEDURES
Valgus Osteotomy to Correct Impingement and Improve Limb Position

Catterall[2] and others have defined methods for managing late femoral head deformity without entering the hip joint. These patients often have pain, a shortened limb, and a limp caused by the coxa vara resulting from severe Perthes disease (**Fig. 2**). These patients sometimes have a flexion contracture with the leg held in adduction to avoid lateral femoral head impingement. Physical examination and radiographic examination can confirm the deformity and cause of symptoms. Often, abducting the hip causes discomfort and pelvic rotation because of the extruded femoral head impinging on the acetabular rim.

Such patients can be improved by extraarticular proximal femoral osteotomies.[3,4] In planning for such an osteotomy, one obtains an adduction radiograph to confirm the position where the more medial portion of the femoral head better centers itself within the acetabulum (**Fig. 3**). An MRI and an arthrogram may also be helpful in this assessment.

In most cases the operative procedure includes a proximal femoral valgus osteotomy, whose

---

The authors have no conflicts of interest or sources of funding to report.
Department of Orthopaedic Surgery, Rady Children's Hospital San Diego, University of California San Diego, 3030 Children's Way, Suite 410, San Diego, CA 92103, USA
* Corresponding author.
E-mail address: orthoedu@rchsd.org

Orthop Clin N Am 42 (2011) 365–372
doi:10.1016/j.ocl.2011.04.009

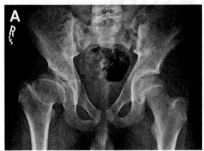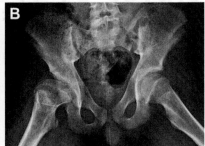

Fig. 1. (*A*) A 14-year-old boy who had Legg-Calvé-Perthes disease at age 8 years and was treated with nonoperative methods. He now has a limp and relatively severe hip pain with activities. (*B*) Frog-leg view in the same patient. This patient typifies the problems encountered in treating the late sequelae of Perthes disease. Treatment choices range from medication and activity restriction to complex osteotomies.

principle is to correct lateral impingement of the femoral head. The extension component of the femoral osteotomy is somewhat less important. The anterolateral impinging portion of the enlarged femoral head is left intact and not removed. This traditional philosophy differs from later treatment ideas, which are presented next, in which the femoral head and neck are recontoured.

Box 1
Surgical approaches for treatment of sequelae of Perthes disease

Extraarticular methods

- Intertrochanteric valgus osteotomy
  - Valgus extension: best corrects limb deformity
  - Valgus flexion: may better correct anterior impingement
- Trochanteric transfer with relative neck lengthening
  - To correct greater trochanteric abutment)
- Noncontainment acetabular procedures
  - Shelf acetabuloplasty
  - Chiari procedure

Intraarticular methods

- Osteochondroplasty of the head and neck (open or via arthroscopy)
  - Note: residual dysplasia may also require treatment
- Femoral head reduction (central "downsizing")
  - Unproved method
- Excision of osteochondritis dissecans
- Labral repair

When significant valgus is performed, the hip is at some risk for instability and in such cases a shelf acetabuloplasty[5,6] can be added to stabilize the hip joint (**Fig. 4**). An added shelf acetabuloplasty supports the labrum and prevents any risk for residual subluxation (**Fig. 5**). Decision regarding which patient should have a valgus osteotomy alone versus which might benefit by the addition of a shelf procedure to prevent femoral head subluxation has not been clearly established and requires experience and judgment.

The overriding principle of extraarticular osteotomy to prevent late deformity in Perthes disease is to reposition the limb so that the child can walk more normally without impinging the lateral segment of the femoral head. At follow-up most patients treated with valgus osteotomy have satisfactory flexion and extension, continued decreased hip rotation, but much improved hip abduction and a significant improvement in limb length difference. Parents and the patient are usually happy with the procedure because of the improvement in functional limb length difference and limp.

Most centers that treat patients with late Perthes disease have had satisfactory results with the procedure and have been slow to move toward femoral head reshaping procedures. One reason for this is that most patients with an enlarged femoral head have some acetabular dysplasia and if the femoral head is brought down to normal size, there is a risk for hip subluxation. Also, there has been less long-term follow-up regarding head–neck reshaping procedures in Perthes disease.

It is important for the surgeon to be aware of gradual knee valgus syndrome (secondary to chronic hip varus). Hip osteotomy can unmask the knee valgus and it may suddenly "appear" following surgery.[7] One may have to warn parents of this phenomenon and may need to perform

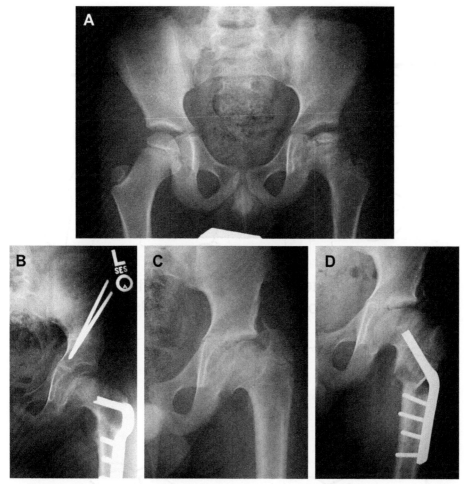

Fig. 2. (A) Left hip Legg-Calvé-Perthes disease in a 10-year-old child. (B) Treatment by combined Salter innominate osteotomy plus femoral varus osteotomy. The femoral head is well-contained. (C) Three years later, the femoral head remains round following containment; however, growth disturbance of the proximal femur caused coxa brevis. The greater trochanter abuts the lateral margin of the acetabulum and limits abduction. (D) Following correction with proximal femoral valgus osteotomy, the hip abduction is improved.

simultaneous medial–distal femoral stapling or acute distal osteotomy or possibly late distal osteotomy.

Greater Trochanteric Transfer (Relative Femoral Neck Lengthening)

Greater-trochanteric abutment is a major problem in many cases of healed Perthes for various reasons. In the nontreated cases it is more likely caused by trochanter overgrowth and relative coax vara with head flattening, whereas in surgically treated cases it is often related to varus osteotomy, which worsens an already existing proximal femoral varus deformity. With better understanding of the proximal femoral vascularity, the position of the soft spot, and subretinacular vessels, relative neck lengthening and trochanteric

distalization[8] have become successful tools in dealing with treatment of mechanical problems of trochanteric abutment and safe-trochanteric distalization.

Acetabular Procedures

It is important to note that true acetabular dysplasia can coexist in cases of Perthes disease as a morphologic response to the flat, elliptical, mushroom-shaped growing femoral head. An important technical point to note is that of potential iatrogenic acetabular undercoverage following femoral procedure, such as open femoral osteo-chondroplasty or head-reduction procedure. These can lead to hip instability caused by the relative imbalance in joint congruity from treating the femoral side and may require an additional

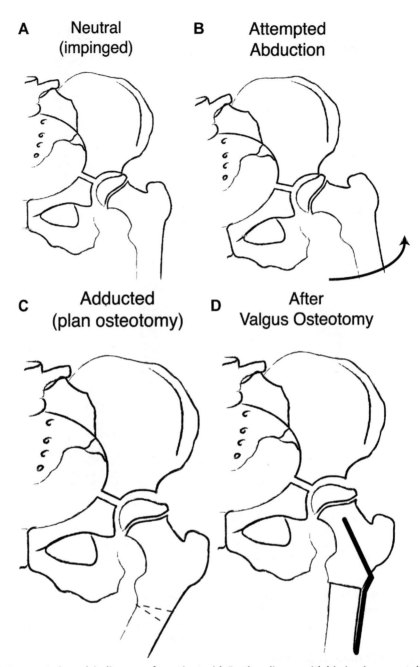

Fig. 3. (*A*) Anteroposterior pelvis diagram of a patient with Perthes disease with hip impingement. (*B*) Attempted abduction causes tilting of the pelvis and hip pain. The lateral portion of the femoral head impinges on the lateral margin of the acetabulum and causes the joint to hinge open medially. (*C*) When planning a valgus osteotomy a radiograph is obtained with the hip in an adducted position to indicate whether the anterolateral bump can be moved away from the acetabular rim. (*D*) Diagram demonstrates correction of impingement and improved pelvic position after proximal femoral valgus osteotomy.

acetabular procedure, such as the Bernese periacetabular osteotomy, to counteract instability.

Other acetabular procedures have also been reported for management of patients with sequelae of Perthes' disease. Shelf acetabuloplasty has

been reported as an alternative to proximal femoral valgus osteotomy for patients who have hinge abduction and severe Perthes disease.[5,9] The Chiari osteotomy has been performed to relieve pain in patients with long-term sequelae

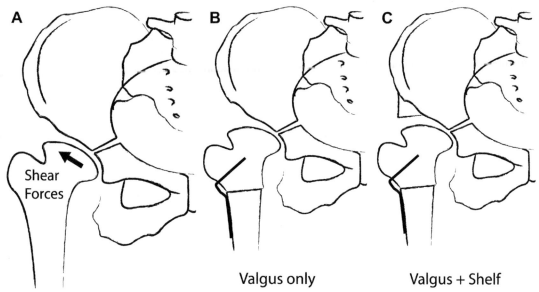

Fig. 4. (*A*) Depiction of femoral head deformity secondary to Perthes with risk for subluxation caused by a dysplastic acetabulum. (*B*) Risk for further subluxation may increase after proximal femoral valgus osteotomy. (*C*) Shelf acetabuloplasty to prevent femoral head migration after proximal femoral valgus osteotomy may be indicated for patients with an upward-sloping acetabular margin.

of Perthes' disease.[10–12] The mechanism for pain relief is uncertain, but there may be an element of labral support and redistribution of weight-bearing forces that improve the mechanics of the hip joint when greater acetabular coverage is obtained. The acetabular dysplasia may need to be addressed in patients with healed Perthes, particularly those that present with typical features of dysplasia, such as sloping acetabular roof, hypertrophied labrum, or large labral tears.

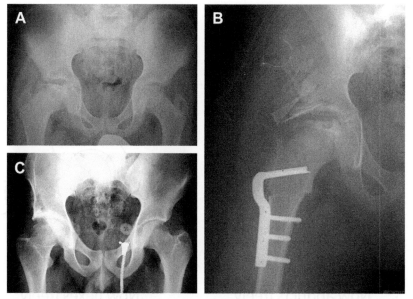

Fig. 5. (*A*) An 11-year-old boy with severe right femoral head deformity caused by Perthes disease. Hinge abduction prevents containment. (*B*) Anteroposterior view of right hip taken intraoperatively after valgus osteotomy plus shelf acetabuloplasty. (*C*) Radiograph obtained 7 years after the surgical procedure. The child is asymptomatic.

INTRAARTICULAR PROCEDURES
Femoral Head–Neck Recontouring Options in Late Healed Perthes Disease

With improved understanding of the vascularity of the proximal femur and the hip joint and the ability safely to dislocate the hip joint after extensive work by Ganz and colleagues,[13] a new era described as "hip preservation" has emerged that can be applied to late, healed Perthes disease.[14]

Intraarticular methods are indicated to address healed Perthes cases with hip impingement (cam, pincer, or mixed). The surgical techniques used can be either the open safe-surgical dislocation with the classic trochanter-flip osteotomy, the anterior arthrotomy technique without hip dislocation, an arthroscopic approach,[15,16] or arthroscopy plus mini-open methods.

The goal of treating cam impingement lesions in the enlarged femoral heads with anterolateral bumps is a well-performed osteochondroplasty of the femoral head–neck junction, to relieve the mechanical abutment that takes place in flexion, adduction, and internal rotation positions of the hip (**Fig. 6**). In cases with mixed impingement the pincer component (caused by retroverted

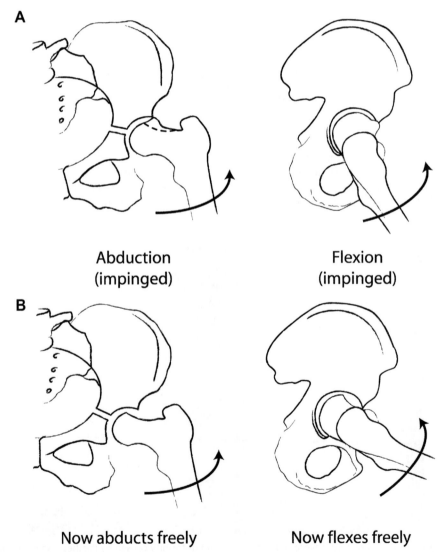

Abduction (impinged)   Flexion (impinged)

Now abducts freely   Now flexes freely

Fig. 6. (A) Diagram of anteroposterior and lateral view of hip with residual Perthes deformity. This illustrates that the impingement may also be anterior with impingement during flexion and abduction. (B) Diagram illustrating osteoplasty or cheilectomy of the femoral head and neck. This can restore motion by removing impingement.

acetabuli, deep acetabuli, or previously failed shelf acetabuloplasty) is managed with an appropriate "rim-trim" or recession with labral reattachment andfixation (**Fig. 7**). The previously mentioned intraarticular methods are reasonably well-documented at this point but not yet confirmed as proved methods.

A more aggressive approach to severe femoral head deformity is the technique of central head reduction that reduces the size of extremely large femoral heads with a saddle shape and central necrosis with depression. In untrained hands these highly technically demanding procedures may be unpredictable.

Arthroscopic osteochondroplasty is possible but technically challenging in cases of Perthes sequelae. Extensive labral takedown and refixation is challenging via the arthroscopic approach.

Also, assessment of residual dysplasia may be more difficult with an arthroscopic-only view point.

Treatment of Osteochondritis Dissecans and Labral Pathology

Osteochondritis dissecans is rare as an isolated cause of late pain following Legg-Calvé-Perthes disease. Symptoms are more commonly caused by deformity of the femoral head with impingement or labral pathology. Treatment of isolated osteochondritis dissecans is usually nonoperative unless the fragment is loose and causing catching or locking of the hip.[17] In these cases it may be possible to remove the fragment arthroscopically. Debridement and repair of labral tears may also relieve pain in some patients but this often needs to be combined with

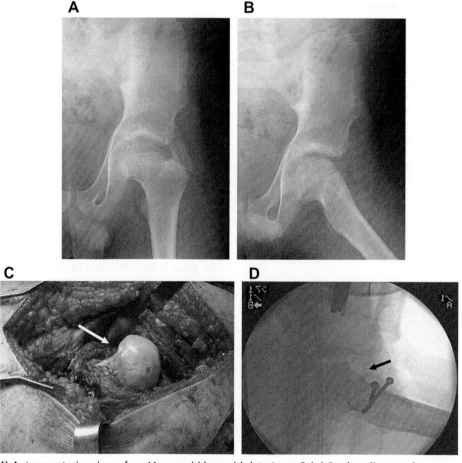

Fig. 7. (A) Anteroposterior view of an 11-year-old boy with late Legg-Calvé-Perthes disease who was previously treated with triple innominate osteotomy, but who now has femoral head impingement and pain. (B) Frog-leg view demonstrating anterofemoral head–neck prominence and lateral acetabular rim impingement. (C) Intraoperative view after open femoral head–neck recontouring (*arrow*) plus trimming of acetabular rim and reattaching labrum (rim-trim). The arrow demonstrates the area where bone has been removed from the anterolateral femoral head neck junction. (D) Frog-leg radiograph demonstrates that the anterolateral impingement has been corrected.

correction of bone deformity to prevent recurrent labral pathology.[16]

SUMMARY

Containment is not a good choice for an incongruent joint and if instability is a component of the disease. In these cases a shelf or Chiari acetabuloplasty may be considered. Other joint preservation methods for older children and teenagers with more severe head involvement include various extraarticular and intraarticular procedures including proximal femoral osteotomy (often valgus), femoral head and neck osteochondroplasty, and femoral head reduction with the addition of acetabular reorientation in some cases. Surgical approaches to residual hip joint deformity in healed Perthes disease will continue to evolve as clinicians gain a further understanding of this fascinating orthopedic disease.

REFERENCES

1. Stulberg SD, Cooperman DR, Wallenstein R. The natural history of Legg-Calve'-Perthes disease. J Bone Joint Surg Am 1981;63:1095.
2. Catterall A. The place of valgus extension femoral osteotomy in the late management of children with Perthes' disease. Ortop Traumatol Rehabil 2004; 6(6):764–9.
3. Myers GJ, Mathur K, O'Hara J. Valgus osteotomy: a solution for late presentation of hinge abduction in Legg-Calve'-Perthes disease. J Pediatr Orthop 2008;28:169–72.
4. Willett K, Hudson I, Catterall A. Lateral shelf acetabuloplasty: an operation for older children with Perthes disease. J Pediatr Orthop 1992;12: 563–8.
5. Staheli LT, Chew DE. Slotted acetabular augmentation in childhood and adolescence. J Pediatr Orthop 1992;12:569–80.
6. Domzalski ME, Glutting J, Bowen JR, et al. Lateral acetabular growth stimulation following a labral support procedure in Legg-Calve-Perthes disease. J Bone Joint Surg Am 2006;88(7):1458–66.
7. Shim JS, Kim HT, Mubarak SJ, et al. Genu valgum in children with coxa vara resulting from hip disease. J Pediatr Orthop 1997;17:225–9.
8. Macnicol MF, Makris D. Distal transfer of the greater trochanter. J Bone Joint Surg Br 1991;73: 838–41.
9. Freeman R, Wainwright AM, Theologis TN, et al. The outcome of patients with hinge abduction in severe Perthes' disease treated by shelf acetabuloplasty. J Pediatr Orthop 2008;28:619–25.
10. Bennett JT, Mazurek RT, Cash JD. Chiari's osteotomy in the treatment of Perthes' disease. J Bone Joint Surg Br 1991;73:225–8.
11. Koyama K, Higuchi F, Inoue A. Modified Chiari osteotomy for arthrosis after Perthes' disease. Acta Orthop Scand 1998;69:129–32.
12. Kotz R, Chiari C, Hofstaetter JG, et al. Long-term experience with Chiari's osteotomy. Clin Orthop Relat Res 2009;467:2215–20.
13. Ganz R, Parvizi J, Beck M, et al. Femoroacetabular impingement: a cause for osteoarthritis of the hip. [review]. Clin Orthop Relat Res 2003;417:112–20.
14. Anderson LA, Erickson JA, Severson EP, et al. Sequelae of Perthes disease: treatment with surgical hip dislocation and relative femoral neck lengthening. J Pediatr Orthop 2010;30(8):758–66.
15. Kocher MS, Kim Y-J, Milllis MB, et al. Hip arthroscopy in children and adolescents. J Pediatr Orthop 2005;25:680–6.
16. Roy D. Arthroscopic findings of the hip in new onset hip pain in adolescents with previous Legg-Calvé-Perthes disease. J Pediatr Orthop B 2005; 14:151–5.
17. Rowe S, Moon ES, Yoon TR, et al. Fate of the osteochondral fragments in osteochondritis dissecans after Legg-Calvé-Perthes' disease. J Bone Joint Surg Br 2001;84:1025–9.

Treatment of Coxa Brevis

Shawn C. Standard, MD

KEYWORDS

- Morscher osteotomy • Coxa brevis • Hip biomechanics
- Proximal femur

The immature proximal femur is a complex structure with a physis that contributes to the shape and relationship of the femoral head, femoral neck, and greater trochanter. Siffert[1] described the complexity of the proximal femoral physis by separating the growth plate into three distinct zones of activity. The three zones consist of the longitudinal growth plate, the femoral neck isthmic growth area, and the trochanteric growth plate (**Fig. 1**).[2] Any disturbance of the normal growth and development of this physis will result in morphologic changes of the proximal femur. A significant shape change of the proximal femur negatively impacts the biomechanics of the hip joint. Altered hip biomechanics result in symptoms of muscle fatigue, pain, and a concurrent limp.[3]

Multiple conditions—including infection, trauma, congenital growth deficiencies or congenital hip dislocation, and avascular necrosis of the femoral epiphysis—can affect the growth and development of the proximal femur. The most common cause of proximal femoral growth disturbance is avascular necrosis of the proximal femoral epiphysis from either an unknown cause, Perthes disease, or from the treatment of congenital hip dislocation. Early in the 1900s, both Waldenström[4] and Perthes[5] described morphologic changes of the femoral neck in patients with avascular necrosis of the femoral epiphysis.[3] Siffert[1] noted that the longitudinal growth plate of the proximal femoral physis depends on the nutrient blood vessels from the femoral epiphysis. Therefore, epiphyseal avascular necrosis of the proximal femoral physis causes an alteration of the longitudinal growth of the femoral neck that allows for a relative "greater trochanteric overgrowth." This results in a foreshortened femoral neck termed coxa brevis (**Fig. 2**).

HIP BIOMECHANICS

A brief review of hip biomechanics during single-leg stance demonstrates the significant effects of coxa brevis on the strength of the hip abductor muscles (gluteus medius and gluteus minimus). During single-leg stance, the hip abductor musculature must generate a force (M) equal or greater than the weight of the body and opposite leg (L) to stabilize the pelvis and to prevent pelvic obliquity or positive Trendelenburg sign. As **Figs. 3** and **4** show, as the femoral neck length increases the hip abductor lever arm increases (Ma). With a longer hip abductor lever arm (Ma), the abductor muscles are more efficient and can counter the weight of the body and opposite limb (L x La) with less force.

Coxa brevis does not only cause a decreased lever arm of the hip, but the relative overgrowth of the greater trochanter decreases the normal tension of the gluteus medius muscle. Elftman[6] demonstrated that the normal muscle tension of

International Center for Limb Lengthening, Rubin Institute for Advanced Orthopedics, Sinai Hospital of Baltimore, 2401 West Belvedere Avenue, Baltimore, MD 21215, USA

E-mail address: sstandard@lifebridgehealth.org

Orthop Clin N Am 42 (2011) 373–387

doi:10.1016/j.ocl.2011.05.002

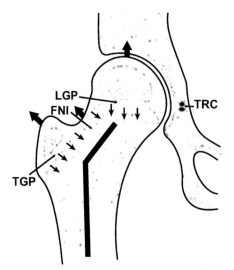

Fig. 1. Siffert's proximal femoral growth plate. The three zones consist of the longitudinal growth plate (LGP), the femoral neck isthmic growth area (FNI), and the trochanteric growth plate (TGP). TRC, triradiate cartilage. (*Adapted from* Stevens PM, Coleman SS. Coxa breva: its pathogenesis and a rationale for its management. J Pediatr Orthop 1985;5(5):515–21; with permission.)

the gluteus medius approaches 0 as the muscle resting length approaches 60% of its normal resting length. The greater trochanteric transfer during the femoral neck-lengthening corrects the tension of the gluteus medius by placing the

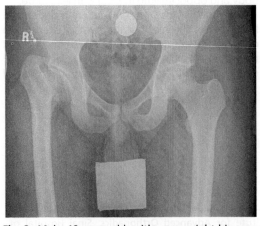

Fig. 2. Male, 19 years old, with severe right-hip coxa brevis after Perthes disease at the age of 6 years. (Copyright 2011, Rubin Institute for Advanced Orthopedics, Sinai Hospital of Baltimore, Baltimore, MD.)

proximal tip of the trochanter at the same level as the center of the femoral head.

RADIOGRAPHIC FINDINGS OF COXA BREVIS

Radiographic evaluation of coxa brevis consists of a supine anteroposterior (AP) and frog lateral view of the pelvis along with a supine AP pelvis with maximum hip adduction of the involved side. The femoral head should be assessed for its shape and congruency within the acetabulum. The scope of this article is limited to coxa brevis with a spherical femoral head and a congruent joint. Basic radiographic measurements should include the neck-shaft angle (NSA), anatomic medial proximal femoral angle (MPFA)[7] (Fig. 5A and B), and the articulotrochanteric distance (ATD) (Fig. 5C and D). In 1965, Edgren[8] described the articulotrochanteric distance (ATD) to objectively quantify the relationship of the femoral head to the greater trochanter (Fig. 5C and D).[1]

By comparing the NSA and the MPFA, one can determine if the proximal femoral deformity is secondary to a coxa vara, coxa brevis, or a combination of the two deformities. This determination allows the surgeon to choose the proper operative technique to correct the deformity.[7] In pure coxa vara, both the NSA and the MPFA will have abnormal values compared with the normal side. However, the amount of difference from the normal value in both the NSA and the MPFA will be equivalent. This situation requires a subtrochanteric valgus osteotomy of the proximal femur (Wagner osteotomy) to correct both the NSA and the MPFA (Fig. 6).

On the other hand, if the preoperative radiograph demonstrates abnormal NSA and MPFA differences that are not equivalent, then a single osteotomy will not correct all components of the proximal femoral deformity (Fig. 7). A better strategy is to perform either a Wagner valgus osteotomy with greater trochanteric transfer or a Morscher femoral neck-lengthening osteotomy (Fig. 8).

When assessing the radiographs of a patient with suspected coxa brevis, the age and skeletal development influences the above described radiographic parameters. Radiographic findings of coxa brevis in a younger patient (<8 years) can be very subtle and include a foreshortened and widened femoral neck as compared with the contralateral side. These findings establish the presence of a proximal femoral growth arrest (Fig. 9). Therefore, it is mandatory to image both hips to allow comparison of the proximal femoral morphology to identify these subtle radiographic findings.

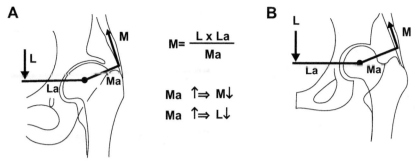

Fig. 3. The biomechanical effects of coxa brevis on the hip joint: L, weight of the body and opposite limb; La, the lever arm of the body; M, the abductor muscular force; and Ma, the lever arm of the hip joint. (*A*) Example of coxa brevis that results in a shortened hip lever arm (Ma). (*B*) Results of a femoral neck-lengthening with an increased hip lever arm (Ma). The increased hip lever arm results in a more efficient hip abductor muscle unit. (*Adapted from* Hasler CC, Morscher EW. Femoral neck-lengthening osteotomy after growth disturbance of the proximal femur. J Pediatr Orthop Part B 1999;8:271–5; with permission.)

Also, the ATD radiographic parameter is inconsistent in younger patients due to the proximal cartilaginous portion of the greater trochanter in patients less than 10 years of age. This creates an apparent ATD versus a true ATD measurement (**Fig. 10**).[3] This inconsistent radiographic parameter makes diagnosis and determination of treatment efficacy in coxa brevis difficult in younger patients. The ATD should be used in patients 10 years of age and older.

To finalize the radiographic assessment of a patient with coxa brevis, bilateral long-standing radiographs should be performed to determine the amount leg-length discrepancy (LLD) that is

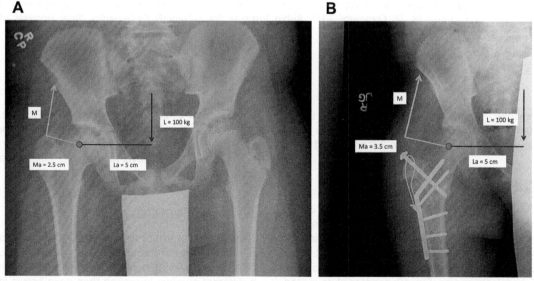

Fig. 4. Preoperative and postoperative: patient with coxa brevis demonstrating the biomechanical effects of the surgical reconstruction. (*A*) The hip abductor muscles must generate force M = 200 kg to counteract the force of the body and left lower limb M = (L × La)/Ma. (*B*) After a femoral neck-lengthening with an increased hip lever arm (Ma), the hip abductor muscles have to generate only a force M = 143 kg to counteract the same force of the body and left lower limb. (Copyright 2011, Rubin Institute for Advanced Orthopedics, Sinai Hospital of Baltimore, Baltimore, MD.)

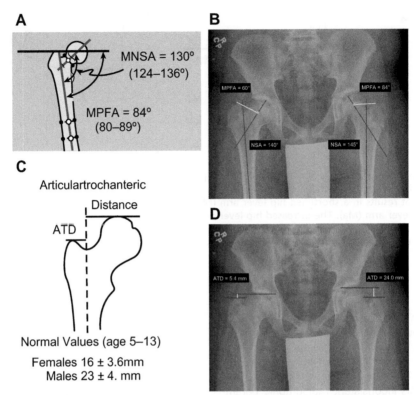

Fig. 5. (*A*) Measurement and population norms for the NSA and the MPFA. (*From* Paley D. Principles of deformity correction. Berlin: Springer-Verlag; 2005; with permission.) (*B*) Coxa brevis with a relative greater trochanteric overgrowth with a normal NSA and an abnormal MPFA as compared with the contralateral side. (*C*) Articulotrochanteric distance (ATD) described by Edgren[5] to objectively determine the relationship between the femoral head and the greater trochanter. Note the population norms for both males and females. (*Adapted from* Stevens PM, Coleman SS. Coxa breva: its pathogenesis and a rationale for its management. J Pediatr Orthop 1985;5(5):515–21; with permission.) (*D*) Objective measurement of the right hip coxa brevis using the ATD described by Edgren.[5] (*B, D*: Copyright 2011, Rubin Institute for Advanced Orthopedics, Sinai Hospital of Baltimore, Baltimore, MD.)

present. Long-standing radiographs usually demonstrate LLD of variable severity. This LLD is usually in the range of 1.5 to 3.0 cm (**Fig. 11**).

CLINICAL FINDINGS OF COXA BREVIS

The clinical findings of coxa brevis include a limping gait, positive Trendelenburg sign, hip impingement and the loss of hip motion. The limping gait results from a combination of the mild LLD and gluteus medius muscle weakness. The positive Trendelenburg sign (**Fig. 12**) denotes gluteus medius weakness or inefficiency as described above in the hip biomechanics section.

Coxa brevis causes hip impingement in both hip abduction and hip rotation. The relative overgrowth of the greater trochanter creates lateral hip impingement in the abducted position (**Fig. 13**). The foreshortened and widened femoral neck can result in anterior impingement with hip flexion and rotation. Coxa brevis also causes loss of hip motion, mainly in the direction of hip abduction.

TREATMENT STRATEGY FOR COXA BREVIS

There are several treatment options for coxa brevis depending on the treatment goals. For example, coxa brevis with a concurrent LLD would require a different surgical approach than coxa brevis in a patient with equal leg lengths. Another variation is the strategy to treat coxa brevis with concurrent femoral acetabular impingement versus a coxa brevis that requires a concurrent change in femoral head position within the acetabulum.

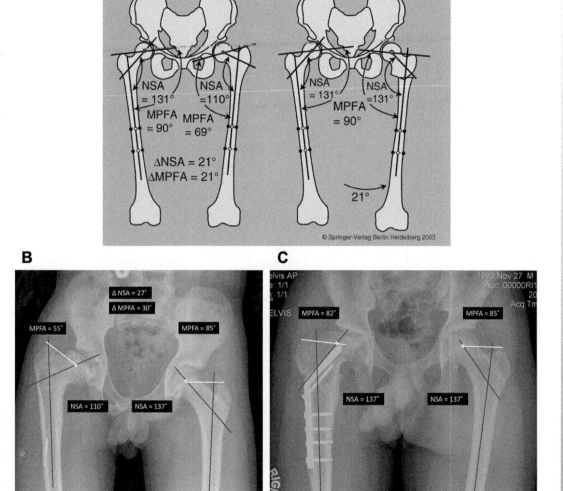

Fig. 6. (*A*) Left hip deformity with abnormal NSA, MPFA, and ATD. However, the quantitative differences of the NSA and MPFA from the contralateral normal side are equal. This denotes a pure coxa vara deformity that can be corrected with a single subtrochanteric valgus osteotomy that corrects all parameters. (*From* Paley D. Principles of deformity correction. Berlin: Springer-Verlag; 2005; with permission.) (*B*) Preoperative: hip with both coxa vara and coxa brevis. However, the quantitative differences of the NSA (27°) and MPFA (30°) are essentially equal. This deformity can be corrected by a single subtrochanteric osteotomy. (*C*) Postoperative: correction of the NSA and MPFA with a subtrochanteric (Wagner) osteotomy. Note the improvement of the lever arm distance of the hip and improved ATD. (*B, C:* Copyright 2011, Rubin Institute for Advanced Orthopedics, Sinai Hospital of Baltimore, Baltimore, MD.)

Coxa Brevis with Concurrent Femoral Acetabular Impingement

The treatment for coxa brevis with concurrent femoral acetabular impingement (FAI) requires an open surgical dislocation with a relative femoral neck-lengthening as described by Eifer and

colleagues.[8] This surgical treatment consists of a surgical dislocation of the hip with excision of bony impingement of the femoral head and neck. As the bony impingement zones are excised, the femoral neck is reshaped using a high speed bur. The greater trochanteric osteotomy performed

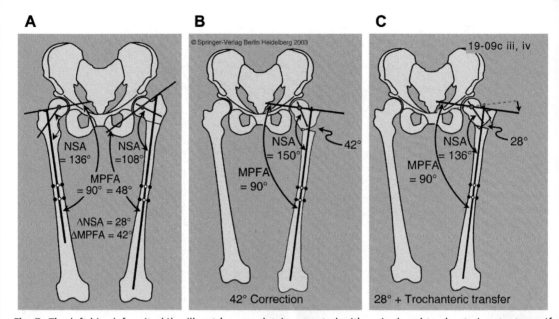

Fig. 7. The left hip deformity (*A*) will not be completely corrected with a single subtrochanteric osteotomy. If a single osteotomy strategy is employed (*B*) and the MPFA normalized, the NSA will be overcorrected to 150°. A better strategy (*C*) is to perform a subtrochanteric osteotomy with a correction of 28° and a separate greater trochanteric osteotomy and transfer distally. (*From* Paley D. Principles of deformity correction. Berlin: Springer-Verlag; 2005; with permission.)

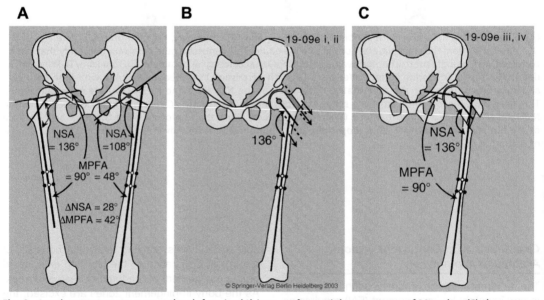

Fig. 8. Another strategy to correct the deformity (*A*) is to perform triple osteotomy of Morscher (*B*) that concurrently lengthens the femoral neck and corrects the proximal femoral deformity (*C*). (*From* Paley D. Principles of deformity correction. Berlin: Springer-Verlag; 2005; with permission.)

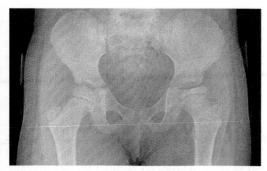

Fig. 9. Female, 6 years old, with findings of initial coxa brevis of the left hip. Note the subtle shortening and widening of the left femoral neck caused by the longitudinal growth disturbance secondary to Perthes disease. (Copyright 2011, Rubin Institute for Advanced Orthopedics, Sinai Hospital of Baltimore, Baltimore, MD.)

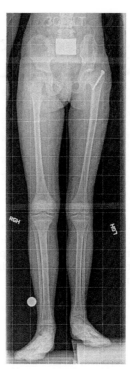

Fig. 11. Female, 10 years old, with left hip coxa brevis and concurrent LLD of 2.5 cm. (Copyright 2011, Rubin Institute for Advanced Orthopedics, Sinai Hospital of Baltimore, Baltimore, MD.)

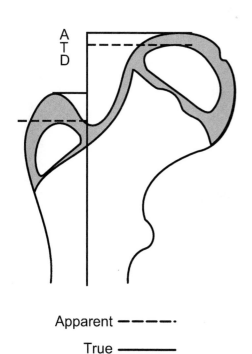

Apparent ----·

True ———

Fig. 10. The cartilaginous portion of the femoral head and greater trochanter in younger patients (<10 years) creates an apparent ATD measurement making diagnosis and treatment efficacy difficult to determine. (*Adapted from* Stevens PM, Coleman SS. Coxa breva: its pathogenesis and a rationale for its management. J Pediatr Orthop 1985;5(5):515–21; with permission.)

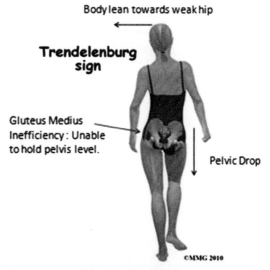

Fig. 12. The positive Trendelenburg sign results in the body lean over the weak hip to counter the pelvic obliquity caused by the weak gluteus medius muscle. (*Courtesy of* Montana Spine and Pain Center, Hamilton, MT; with permission.)

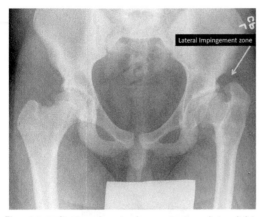

Fig. 13. Left coxa brevis demonstrating lateral hip impingement with loss of hip abduction due to greater trochanter overgrowth. (Copyright 2011, Rubin Institute for Advanced Orthopedics, Sinai Hospital of Baltimore, Baltimore, MD.)

for the surgical dislocation is repaired with a concurrent advancement of the greater trochanter. This results in the relative lengthening of the femoral neck with improvement of the hip's lever arm (**Fig. 14**).

Coxa Brevis with Equal Leg Lengths

The treatment of coxa brevis in a patient with equal leg lengths requires an isolated greater trochanteric advancement (**Fig. 15**). A detailed radiographic and clinical examination is needed to insure that concurrent FAI, LLD, or coxa vara is not present. The isolated greater trochanteric advancement represents a relative femoral neck-lengthening as described above.

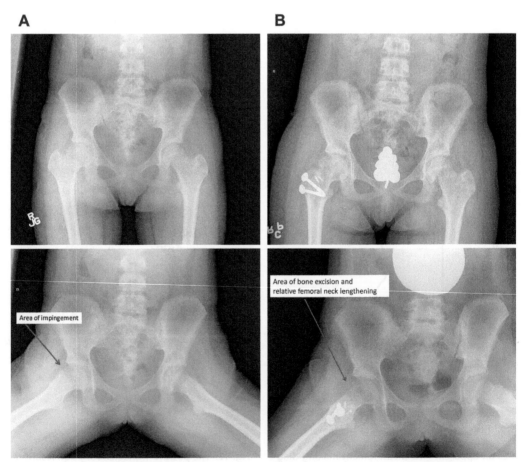

Fig. 14. (A) Female, 13 years old, 5 years after hip distraction treatment for a Herring C stage Perthes disease with recurrent pain secondary to anterior hip impingement. (B) Postoperative: surgical dislocation of the hip demonstrating the anterior impingement excision and relative femoral neck-lengthening with greater trochanteric advancement. (Copyright 2011, Rubin Institute for Advanced Orthopedics, Sinai Hospital of Baltimore, Baltimore, MD.)

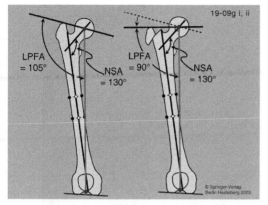

Fig. 15. Isolated coxa brevis or relative trochanteric overgrowth corrected with a greater trochanteric advancement. LPFA, lateral proximal femoral angle. (*From* Paley D. Principles of deformity correction. Berlin: Springer-Verlag; 2005; with permission.)

Coxa Brevis with Concurrent LLD

Coxa brevis with concurrent LLD can be corrected using one of two strategies. Both strategies result in lengthening of the involved extremity; however,

the relationship of the femoral head relative to the acetabulum changes with the first strategy and remains the same with the second strategy.

The first surgical strategy is a valgus osteotomy at the subtrochanteric level with or without a concurrent advancement of the greater trochanter. This procedure is commonly known as the Wagner osteotomy and demonstrated in **Fig. 6**. This surgical strategy is used when a true coxa vara and coxa brevis are present in the proximal femur and the femoral head is more congruent when the hip is adducted (**Fig. 16**).

The second surgical strategy is a true femoral neck-lengthening with a greater trochanteric transfer performed via three parallel osteotomies. The femoral head relationship to the acetabulum is unchanged. This procedure is commonly known as the Morscher osteotomy and is the subject of interest for the remainder of this article.

MORSCHER OSTEOTOMY
Indications

The Morscher osteotomy is indicated in a patient with coxa brevis, a congruent hip joint, and a LLD of 2 to 3 cm. Coxa vara is not a contraindication to this type of femoral neck-lengthening. The

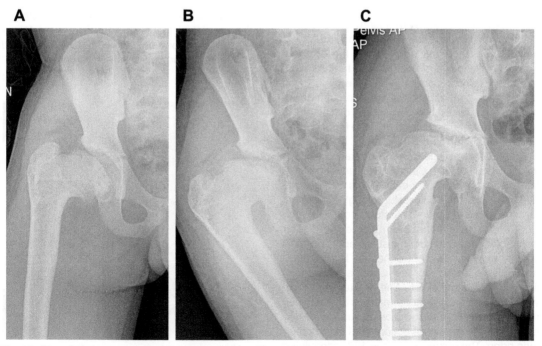

A **B** **C**

Fig. 16. (*A* and *B*) Preoperative: male, 14 years old, with a previous varus osteotomy. Neutral and adducted anteroposterior (AP) view of the hip. The adducted view allows the relationship of the femoral head to the acetabulum to be determined before the valgus osteotomy. (*C*) Postoperative: final position of the femoral head after the valgus osteotomy. (Copyright 2011, Rubin Institute for Advanced Orthopedics, Sinai Hospital of Baltimore, Baltimore, MD.)

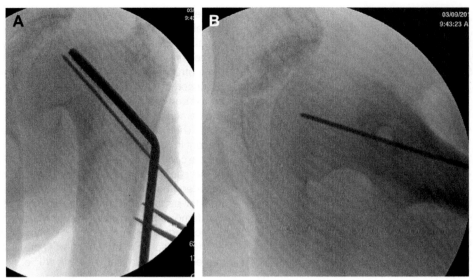

Fig. 17. (*A* and *B*) Guidewire inserted in the center of the femoral neck in AP and lateral views. Note in the AP view the cannulated blade plate is being held anterior to the thigh to check the ankle of guidewire insertion. (Copyright 2011, Rubin Institute for Advanced Orthopedics, Sinai Hospital of Baltimore, Baltimore, MD.)

neck shaft angle is corrected by adjusting the angle of the subtrochanteric osteotomy and is described below.

Surgical Technique

Additional preoperative radiographic measurements should include the length and width of the femoral neck and the diameter of the proximal femur. The length and width of the femoral neck will determine the correct size blade plate to be used for the surgical procedure. The diameter of the proximal femur will be used to calculate the amount of lateral displacement of the femoral shaft that will be performed.

The patient is placed on the operating table in a supine position with a small bump under the ipsilateral sacrum. The lower extremity is widely prepped to include the iliac crest, groin, gluteal region, and the entire lower limb. A standard lateral incision is created starting 2 cm above the greater trochanter and extending distally approximately 10 cm below the greater trochanter. The subcutaneous tissue and tensor fascia lata are divided in line with the skin incision. The greater trochanter with the attached gluteus medius is identified and the vastus lateralis muscle is subperiosteally elevated in an anterior direction off of the trochanteric ridge. The guidewire for the 130° cannulated blade plate (custom device from Smith and Nephew, Memphis, TN, USA) is inserted in the center of the femoral neck under fluoroscopic guidance (**Fig. 17**).

The guidewire is inserted at an angle of 130° to match the angle of the blade plate and to create a normal neck shaft angle. Three additional guidewires are inserted parallel to the femoral neck guidewire marking the three osteotomies of the Morscher procedure (**Fig. 18**). The three osteotomies consist of the greater trochanteric osteotomy, the superior femoral neck osteotomy, and the inferior femoral neck osteotomy.

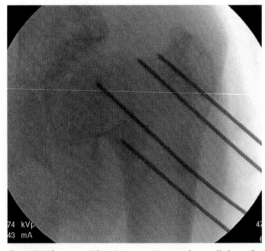

Fig. 18. Three guidewires are inserted parallel to the initial femoral neck wire; the three osteotomies of the Morscher procedure. (Copyright 2011, Rubin Institute for Advanced Orthopedics, Sinai Hospital of Baltimore, Baltimore, MD.)

A large sagittal saw is used and the greater trochanteric osteotomy is performed using the most superior wire as a guide. The greater trochanteric fragment with the attached gluteus medius muscle is mobilized with careful dissection. The second osteotomy along the superior femoral neck guidewire is performed creating a block of free bone graft. This bone block is very important and must be saved to be used as the lateral graft (**Fig. 19**). **Technical tip: for the second cut, use a curved osteotome after the sagittal saw to complete the osteotomy. The curve of the osteotome is pointed superiorly to produce an improved contour of the superior femoral neck (Fig. 20).**

The cannulated chisel is used to create a path for the cannulated blade plate over the initial femoral guide wire. **Technical tip: insure that no flexion or extension is created by keeping the inferior chisel surface in line with the femoral shaft.** When the chisel is fully seated, the length of the blade plate is calculated by adding 10 to 15 mm to the chisel length that is inside the femoral neck. The exact amount of blade plate

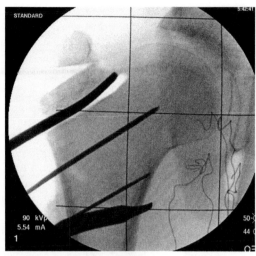

Fig. 20. A curved osteotome is used to complete the osteotomy initiated by the sagittal saw to reproduce the superior femoral neck contour. (Copyright 2011, Rubin Institute for Advanced Orthopedics, Sinai Hospital of Baltimore, Baltimore, MD.)

left exposed represents the amount of lateral translation that will occur when the final inferior femoral neck osteotomy is performed. The amount of lateral translation should not exceed one half of the measured diameter of the proximal femur. With the cannulated chisel fully seated in the femoral neck, the final inferior femoral neck osteotomy is performed with the sagittal saw (**Fig. 21**). This

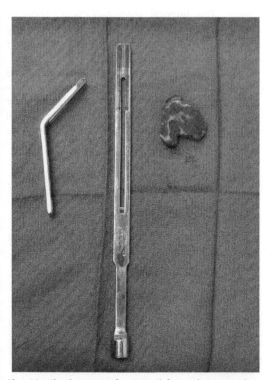

Fig. 19. The bone graft created from the second osteotomy with the cannulated blade plate and cannulated chisel. (Copyright 2011, Rubin Institute for Advanced Orthopedics, Sinai Hospital of Baltimore, Baltimore, MD.)

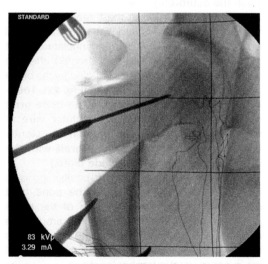

Fig. 21. Intraoperative: the final inferior femoral neck osteotomy. (Copyright 2011, Rubin Institute for Advanced Orthopedics, Sinai Hospital of Baltimore, Baltimore, MD.)

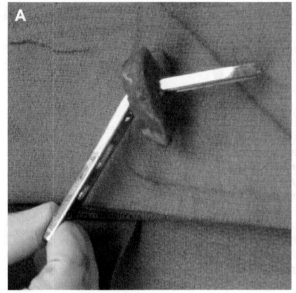
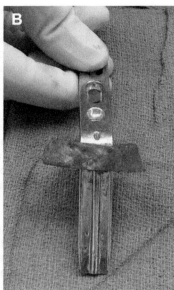

Fig. 22. (*A* and *B*) The bone graft segment is placed over the blade plate before insertion of the cannulated blade plate over the initial guidewire. (Copyright 2011, Rubin Institute for Advanced Orthopedics, Sinai Hospital of Baltimore, Baltimore, MD.)

cut is parallel to the guidewire and re-establishes a neck shaft angle of 130°. **Technical tip: while performing this osteotomy, use the chisel as a handle and gently open the osteotomy site by levering the chisel proximally. The surgeon must remember to follow the guidewire or chisel in the femoral neck and remain parallel to it as the pressure on the chisel wedges open the osteotomy site.**

After the completion of the three osteotomies, the cannulated chisel is removed from the femoral neck and replaced with the cannulated blade plate. The bone graft segment created after the second osteotomy should be impaled by the blade plate before blade plate insertion (**Fig. 22**). **Technical tip: drill multiple holes in the bone graft segment with a 1.5 to 2.0 Kirschner wire at the area of blade plate placement. Gently create an opening in the bone graft with the chisel and then insert the blade plate.**)

Another option for bone graft positioning is to create a "keyhole" opening in the bone graft segment (**Fig. 23**). After insertion of the blade plate, place the prepared bone graft around the exposed portion of the blade. The bone graft is stabilized by the "press fit" around the blade and the eventual greater trochanter repair.

After the blade plate is fully seated into the chisel path, a bone reduction clamp is used to reduce the femoral shaft to the plate and secured with cortical screws. The femoral shaft reduction produces lateral translation of the distal segment, thereby lengthening the femoral neck and the lower extremity (**Fig. 24**).

The final step is the reduction and fixation of the greater trochanter. The greater trochanteric fragment is first advanced distally until the superior tip of the trochanter is located at the same level as the center of the femoral head. The greater

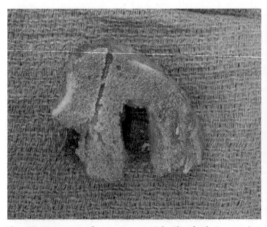

Fig. 23. Bone graft segment with "keyhole" opening for placement over the inserted blade plate. (Copyright 2011, Rubin Institute for Advanced Orthopedics, Sinai Hospital of Baltimore, Baltimore, MD.)

A

B

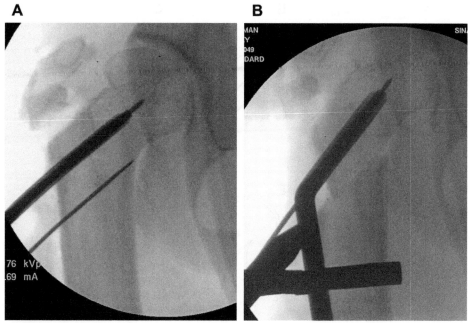

Fig. 24. Intraoperative: (*A*) femoral shaft before subtrochanteric osteotomy and (*B*) the femoral shaft being reduced to the plate creating a lateral translation and femoral neck-lengthening. (Copyright 2011, Rubin Institute for Advanced Orthopedics, Sinai Hospital of Baltimore, Baltimore, MD.)

trochanter is temporarily secured with a Kirschner wire and its position confirmed under fluoroscopy **Technical tip: place the hip in moderate abduction to allow the trochanteric fragment to be advanced distally without undue tension).** The greater trochanteric advancement is then secured with a 5.5 mm cannulated screw (Smith and Nephew) and a tension band wire (**Fig. 25**).

A summary of the surgical technique is demonstrated in schematic form in **Fig. 26** and a radiographic example is demonstrated in **Fig. 27**.

Postoperative Care

Postoperatively, the patient is placed in a single-leg hip abduction orthosis that is worn full time except for showering. The patient remains in the brace and is allowed only toe-touch weight-bearing for the first 6 weeks. During this initial period, physical therapy consists of gentle passive hip range of motion in abduction (30°), flexion (90°), extension (full), and rotation (not greater than 30°). At 6 weeks postoperatively, the hip abduction orthosis is worn only at night and the patient advances to full weight-bearing under physical therapist guidance. During physical therapy, active and passive hip range of motion is performed in all directions along with strengthening. At 3 months postoperatively, the patient

is brace-free and fully weight-bearing. Therapy continues until the patient regains hip range of motion and strength that allows for normal gait and function.

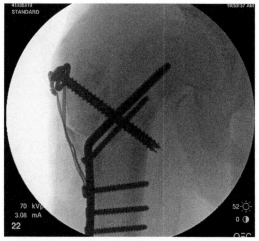

Fig. 25. Completion of the procedure with advancement and fixation of the greater trochanteric fragment using a 5.5 mm cannulated screw and tension band wire. (Copyright 2011, Rubin Institute for Advanced Orthopedics, Sinai Hospital of Baltimore, Baltimore, MD.)

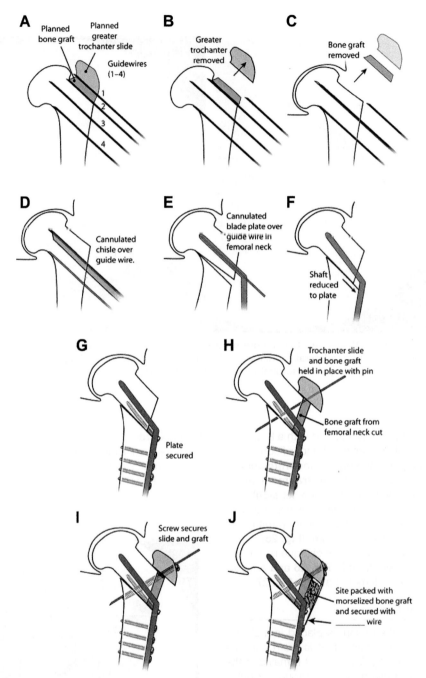

Fig. 26. Morscher osteotomy. (Copyright 2011, Rubin Institute for Advanced Orthopedics, Sinai Hospital of Baltimore, Baltimore, MD.)

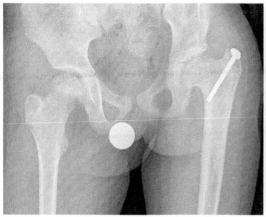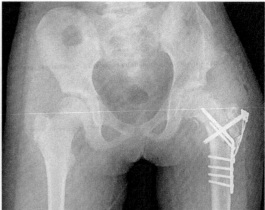

Fig. 27. Preoperative and postoperative: Morscher osteotomy on female, 12 years old. (Copyright 2011, Rubin Institute for Advanced Orthopedics, Sinai Hospital of Baltimore, Baltimore, MD.)

SUMMARY

Coxa brevis of the hip results in a significant morphologic change of the proximal femur that creates a poor mechanical environment for the hip joint. This proximal femoral deformity creates pain, fatigue, LLD, and an altered gait in the affected patient. The most common cause of coxa brevis is a growth alteration of the proximal femoral physis secondary to ischemic necrosis of the proximal femoral epiphysis. In 1980, Dr Erwin Morscher developed a unique femoral neck-lengthening technique that afforded both correction of the proximal femoral deformity and the LLD. Both preliminary and long-term reviews of this procedure have demonstrated the significant benefit of restoring the proper biomechanics of the hip with concurrent leg-length equalization.[2,9,10] In my personal experience, the Morscher osteotomy is a very successful and predictable surgical technique for the treatment of coxa brevis with concurrent LLD. My patients have uniformly experienced significant improvement in gait and hip abductor strength. In addition, the symptoms of fatigue and hip discomfort resolve. I have not experienced any occurrences of nonunion, infection, or hardware failure. The average leg-length gain has been 1.7 cm in my patients undergoing a femoral neck-lengthening osteotomy. The Morscher osteotomy as described above restores the normal proximal femur morphology and biomechanics resulting in successful treatment of coxa brevis.

REFERENCES

1. Siffert R. Patterns of deformity in the developing hip. Clin Orthop 1981;160:14–29.
2. Schneidmueller D, Carstens C, Thomsen M. Surgical treatment of overgrowth of the greater trochanter in children and adolescents. J Pediatr Orthop 2006; 26(4):486–90.
3. Stevens PM, Coleman SS. Coxa breva: its pathogenesis and a rationale for its management. J Pediatr Orthop 1985;5(5):515–21.
4. Waldenström H. Die Tuberkulose des Collum Femoris im Kindesalter und ihre Beziehungen zur Hüftgelenkentzündung. Stockholm, Norstedt; 1910.
5. Edgren W. Coxa plana. Acta Orthop Scand Suppl 1965;84:1–129.
6. Elftman H. Biomechanics of muscle. J Bone Joint Surg Am 1966;48:363–77.
7. Paley D. Principles of deformity correction. 1st edition, Corr. 2nd printing. Berlin: Springer-Verlag; 2003.
8. Eifer H, Podeszwar DA, Ganz R, et al. Evaluation and treatment of young adults with femoro-acetabular impingement secondary to Perthes' disease. Hip Int 2006;16(4):273–80.
9. Hasler CC, Morscher EW. Femoral neck lengthening osteotomy after growth disturbance of the proximal femur. J Pediatr Orthop B 1999;8:271–5.
10. Buess P, Morscher E. Osteotomy to lengthen the femur neck with distal adjustment of the trochanter major in coxa vara after hip dislocation. Orthopade 1988;17:485–90.

The Treatment of Femoral Head Deformity and Coxa Magna by the Ganz Femoral Head Reduction Osteotomy

Dror Paley, MD, FRCSC

KEYWORDS

- Femoral head deformity • Coxa magna • Ganz osteotomy
- Femoral head reduction

Perthes disease often results in a nonspherical femoral head (coxa plana) that is enlarged (coxa magna) compared with the normal side, with a short femoral neck (coxa breva) and a relatively high greater trochanter (coxa vara). The femoral head shape can vary from spherical to ellipsoid, to cylindrical, to saddle shaped. The acetabulum may also change in shape[1] conforming to the enlarged, flattened femoral head or becoming more dysplastic in reaction to the subluxed femoral head. The femoral head cartilage may be well preserved or degenerated. Degeneration of the femoral head cartilage is usually greatest in relation to the rim of the acetabulum. The rim of the acetabulum acts as a high concentration stress line that leads to indentation of the softened femoral head, contributing to the collapse of the femoral head. The cartilage along this indented part of the femoral head may become permanently concave as part of a saddle shaped femoral head. The best-preserved cartilage of the femoral head is often the lateral third, because this part of the head is permanently outside of the joint and experiences little wear and tear and no weight-bearing forces. Similarly, the medial cartilage of the femoral head is often well preserved because of the containment by the round acetabulum. The better molded the two are to each other (congruity), the less wear and degeneration in the medial third of the femoral head.

The treatment of Perthes disease can be divided into 4 time frames: precollapse; collapsed but not ossified; collapsed and ossified; remodeled and degenerative. Treatment during precollapse includes modalities to prevent collapse and speed reossification (bisphosphonates,[2] core decompression,[3] and containment methods[4]). Treatment after collapse but before reossification aims at reduction of the subluxation, restoration of range of motion, and molding of the femoral head to the acetabulum (containment methods using casting and/or osteotomy and soft tissue releases,[5,6] and hip joint distraction[7]). Treatment after the femoral head is collapsed and ossified is aimed at reducing femoroacetabular impingement and at eliminating secondary deformities such as fixed flexion and adduction of the hip joint (valgus osteotomy[8] and femoral head reshaping[9–17]). Finally, once the femoral head and the acetabulum have remodeled fully, incongruity and femeroacetabular impingement leads to degenerative changes of the cartilage of the femoral head and acetabulum. Treatment during this phase ranges from femoral head reshaping,[16,17] hip arthrodesis,[18] pelvis support osteotomy,[19] and prosthetic joint replacement.[20]

The prognosis in Perthes disease is very strongly correlated with the final shape of the femoral head.[21–23] The Stulberg classification[23] of the femoral head is the most prognostic indicator of

Paley Advanced Limb Lengthening Institute, 901 45th Street, West Palm Beach, FL 33407, USA
E-mail address: dpaley@lengthening.us

Orthop Clin N Am 42 (2011) 389–399
doi:10.1016/j.ocl.2011.04.006

longevity of the femoral head. Although painful degenerative changes of the femoral head leading to the need for joint replacement are the final outcome of most Stulberg 4 and 5 hips, femeroacetabular impingement is a probably much earlier and more common problem with Perthes hips including Stulberg 2, 3, 4, and 5. Reshaping of the femoral head with cheilectomy has met with variable success.[9–14] Long-term follow-up of cheilectomy done prior to the recent surgical dislocation approach shows good short-term improvement but no alteration in the degenerative natural history of the disease.[15] The recent introduction of new methods to evaluate, understand, and treat the impingement of the misshapen femoral head has led to a renaissance of interest in the treatment of late Perthes disease. The older procedure of cheilectomy of the femoral head has been replaced by arthroscopic or open osteochondroplasty of the femoral head.[14,16,17,24] The feared complication of avascular necrosis (AVN) of the femoral head has been reduced by the "safe surgical dislocation method" introduced by Reinhold Ganz.[25] This approach has permitted more aggressive and extensive safe resection of the enlarged, impinging portions of the femoral head, with restoration of spherical congruity and movement of the hip joint.

In 2001 Ganz and colleagues[16,17] developed a new solution to the misshapen femoral head of Perthes disease. Ganz recognized that the central third of the enlarged femoral head was the most damaged while the lateral third had the best preservation of cartilage, as already explained. He therefore resected the central third of the femoral head while preserving and mobilizing the vascular pedicle to the lateral third. The resection of the central third was also done in a way to preserve the vascular pedicle to the medial third of the femoral head. After resecting the lateral third he advanced it to the medial third. Essentially, he removed the central part of an ellipsoid and brought the two spherical hemispheric ends together to reform a sphere. He called this femoral head reduction osteotomy (FHRO).[16,17] This intra-articular osteotomy of the femoral head was stabilized with internal fixation screws.

The author has been performing the intra-articular FHRO since February 2006. The purpose of this article is to report the results of the author's first 20 patients to undergo this procedure.

PATIENTS AND METHODS

Between February 2006 and February 2010, 21 patients with misshapen femoral heads underwent intra-articular FHRO to reshape the femoral head. One of these patients suffered a femoral neck fracture in surgery, resulting in conversion to a total hip replacement. This patient was eliminated from the study, leaving 20 patients between 1 and 5 years since the osteotomy (mean 2.7 years). The etiology of the femoral head pathology was Perthes in 15, adolescent AVN in 3, and dysplasia in 2 (**Table 1**). This study comprises a retrospective follow-up of the radiographs and clinical notes of this group of patients. Fourteen patients were treated for the right hip and 6 for the left hip. There were 8 males and 12 females. The average age at the time of the osteotomy was 14 years (range 10–23 years). Five patients were skeletally mature at the time of the osteotomy. In the rest the femoral head physis was still open on the treatment side In only one.

All patients complained of preoperative pain, which was attributed to femoroacetabular impingement, abductor muscle fatigue, or hip joint degeneration. All of the patients had evidence of limp, frequently including a lurch component, antalgic component, and a leg length discrepancy component. All patients had a positive acute or delayed Trendelenburg sign. Range of motion of the hip was reduced in all patients but was considered very stiff in 8 preoperatively. The rest had good preservation of flexion and extension range of the hip joint, with varying degrees of loss of passive abduction and rotation motion of the hip joint.

Four cases were bilateral but only had the osteotomy performed on one side at the time of this study. The other side is being considered for the same treatment but has not yet undergone surgery. Radiographic examination included measurement of the maximum anteroposterior (AP) diameter of the femoral head before and after the head reduction in all patients, and comparison with the normal other side in the 16 unilateral cases. In 4 of the cases the femoral head shape was also altered on the frog lateral or cross-table lateral radiograph of the hip.

Treatment alternatives were discussed with all patients as part of the informed consent process, including valgus intertrochanteric osteotomy, surgical dislocation with cheilectomy, hip fusion, pelvic support osteotomy, and hip replacement.

SURGICAL METHOD

The technique used is modified from that recently published by Ganz and colleagues (**Fig. 1**).[16,17] The patient is positioned in the lateral decubitus position with the affected side up. After prepping and draping the patient with the leg free, a bump is placed to abduct the leg. A midlateral incision from just distal to the iliac crest to a handbreadth

Table 1
Cases of patients with misshapen femoral heads who underwent intra-articular femoral head reduction osteotomy (February 2006 to February 2010)

Patient	Age (y)	Sex	Diagnosis	Bilateral	% Pre	% Other Pre	% Other Post	Year/ Month	AVN	ROM Pre	ROM Post	Pain Post	Gait Post	Result	Pelvis Osteotomy	Follow-Up (y)	EF	Biplanar
1	12	F	Dysplasia	Yes	72	—	—	2006/4	—	—	More	—	Better	E	Yes	5	—	—
2	16	M	AVN	—	87	115	92	2006/7	—	—	More	—	Better	E	—	5	—	—
3	20	F	Perthes	Yes	81	—	—	2006/9	—	—	More	—	Better	E	Yes	4.5	—	—
4	14	M	Perthes	—	71	140	100	2008/4	—	—	More	—	Better	E	—	3	—	Yes
5	11	F	Perthes	—	84	125	95	2008/4	—	—	More	—	Better	E	—	4	Yes	—
6	11	M	Perthes	—	70	150	100	2007/10	—	—	More	—	Better	G	—	3.6	—	—
7	15	F	Perthes	—	88	118	92	2007/10	—	Stiff	Stiff	—	Better	P	—	3.4	—	—
8	10	M	Perthes	—	57	160	84	2008/3	—	Stiff	More	Yes	Better	G	—	3	Yes	—
9	21	M	Perthes	—	67	150	100	2008/9	—	Stiff	More	—	Better	G	—	2.5	—	Yes
10	23	F	AVN	—	83	118	91	2008/5	—	—	More	—	Better	E	—	3.1	—	—
11	13	F	Perthes	—	80	119	100	2008/2	—	—	More	—	Better	E	—	3	—	—
12	11	M	Perthes	Yes	77	—	—	2009/6	—	—	More	—	Better	G	—	2.9	—	—
13	11	M	Perthes	Yes	62	—	—	2009/6	AVN	—	More	—	Better	P	Yes	2	Yes	Yes
14	11	F	Perthes	—	70	141	100	2009/9	—	Stiff	Stiff	Yes	Better	P	Yes	1.5	Yes	—
15	13	M	Perthes	—	72	120	100	2010/4	—	Stiff	More	Yes	Better	G	—	1	—	—
16	17	M	Dysplasia	—	67	127	100	2010/11	—	Stiff	More	—	Better	G	Yes	1	Yes	Yes
17	13	M	Perthes	—	81	150	91	2008/9	—	—	Stiff	—	Better	G	—	2.5	—	—
18	13	M	Perthes	—	76	129	93	2008/9	—	Stiff	Stiff	—	Better	G	—	2.5	—	—
19	18	F	AVN	—	76	132	100	2009/10	—	Stiff	More	—	Better	G	—	1.5	—	—
20	12	M	Perthes	—	82	140	100	2009/10	—	—	Stiff	—	Better	G	—	1.5	—	—
Mean	14	—	—	—	75	133	96	—	—	Stiff	—	—	—	—	—	2.7	—	—

Abbreviations: AVN, avascular necrosis; E, excellent; EF, external fixator; G, good; P, poor; Post, postoperative; Pre, preoperative; ROM, range of motion.

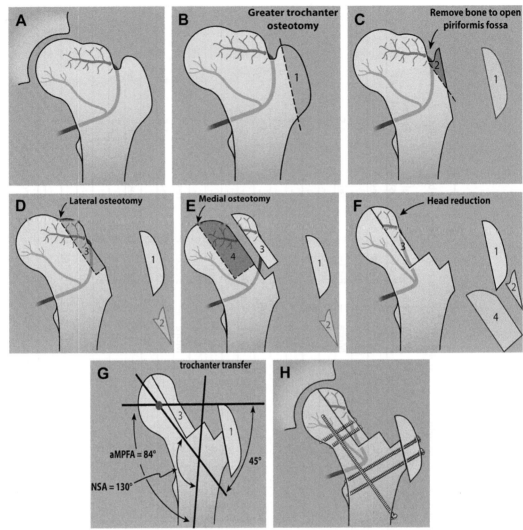

Fig. 1. Femoral head reduction osteotomy (FHRO) technique. (*A*) Coxa magna with saddle-shaped femoral head. The lateral retinacular and the medial branch of the medial femoral circumflex artery are shown. (*B*) Surgical dislocation is performed after a trochanteric flip osteotomy. (*C*) The medial part of the stable trochanter is resected to decompress and mobilize the piriformis fossa and the retinacular pedicular flap. (*D*) The lateral femoral head osteotomy is performed, preserving its vascular pedicle. (*E*) The medial femoral head osteotomy is performed and the segment of the femoral head resected. (*F*) The lateral segment is advanced and fixed to the medial part of the femoral head. (*G*) A relative neck lengthening is achieved by transferring the trochanter distally and laterally. The goal is to achieve normal joint orientation and for the tip of the greater trochanter to be at the level of the center of the femoral head. aMPFA, anatomic proximal femoral shaft angle; NSA, neck shaft angle. (*H*) Headless screws are used to fix the femoral head and neck. Screws with washers are used to fix the greater trochanter.

distal to the greater trochanter is made to and through the fascia lata. The fascia lata is separated from the gluteus maximus muscle anteriorly until the intermuscular septum with the tensor fascia lata is reached. The gluteus maximus muscle is then mobilized from the septum and retracted posteriorly. The hip is then internally rotated. The piriformis tendon and muscle are identified at the posterior border of the gluteus medius and minimus muscles. A retractor is inserted between the hip capsule and the gluteus minimus. The vastus lateralis is elevated off of the proximal femur and retracted with a Homan retractor. The femur is internally rotated to expose the posterior part of the greater trochanter, so that a saw can be properly rotated to perform the trochanteric osteotomy while also clearing the posterior skin and soft tissues. The line connecting the elevated vastus and glutei is visualized and the greater trochanter is osteotomized with a saw along this line, staying lateral to the piriformis tendon. The partial-thickness segment of greater trochanter remains attached to the gluteus minimus, gluteus medius, and vastus lateralis muscles. The piriformis tendon is often split by the osteotomy, with part of it remaining attached to the more medial stable trochanter and part to the mobile trochanteric segment. The piriformis fibers are released off of the mobile trochanter. The mobile trochanter is flipped anteriorly with its trigastric muscles (gluteus medius, gluteus minimus, and vastus lateralis). The gluteus minimus muscle should be reflected off of the capsule and supra-acetabular ileum. One Homan retractor should be hammered into this bone proximal to the acetabulum and one should be inserted over the anterior inferior spine. The reflected tendon of the rectus femoris can be either left alone or released and reflected anteriorly as needed. The hip can now be externally rotated to tension and expose the capsule. The capsulotomy is made in a Z-shaped manner. The transverse limb is made at 1 or 11 o'clock on the right and left hips, respectively, from lateral to medial, without cutting the labrum. The longitudinal arms of the Z should be anterior lateral along the lateral aspect of the neck going distally and posterior along the acetabular rim medially. The femur can be externally rotated while dropping the leg and knee over the anterior side of the table into a sterile pocket. In doing so, the femoral head will start to dislocate. The ligamentum teres may restrict the dislocation and should be cut with long curved type of scissors to release the femoral head from the acetabulum. The femoral head is now fully dislocated and can be inspected circumferentially. The areas of degeneration of cartilage can be identified. The acetabulum can also be inspected and probed to look for cartilage and labral tears. Labral tears should be repaired with sutures. Cartilage flaps should be debrided. Microfracture can be done to any denuded cartilage areas. In children this is not commonly the situation. The ligamentum teres should be resected from the femoral head and from the depth of the acetabulum. The femoral head shape can now be measured with a femoral head spherical template (Wright Medical, Memphis, TN, USA). The most important measurement is the spherical size of the medial femoral head. Medial-lateral and anterior-posterior measurements are taken. This portion of the femoral head is the part that has remained articulating in the acetabulum. It is therefore the right size and shape. The lateral part of the femoral head can also be template with the femoral head spherical templates. Finally, the acetabulum should be templated using the ball-shaped templates from a total hip replacement instrumentation set. The femoral head spherical template is used in a medial-lateral direction to see where the femoral head leaves the round. This point is marked with a pen. The femoral head can now be reduced into the acetabulum. It should be observed for impingement with the acetabulum by taking it through different ranges of motion (flexion, flexion-internal rotation, abduction in flexion and extension). While the femoral head is reduced again, the stable trochanter should be resected to decompress and expose the vessels to the femoral head. The line of resection should follow the physis of the greater trochanter in children. The osteotome should cut from lateral to medial and distal to proximal, and from anterior to posterior. The osteotome should not penetrate the piriformis fossa posteromedially. It should crack the medial cortex and then using a knife, and a pituitary clamp for traction, the bone fragment should be peeled away from the medial soft tissues. Anteriorly, less bone is removed while posteriorly, resection of bone is more distal, paralleling the increasing depth of the piriformis fossa posteriorly. The medial soft tissues should not be disturbed. The hip can be redislocated after the resection of the stable trochanter. The next step is to decide on the osteotomy lines. Two osteotomies are made, one medial and one lateral, resecting a segment of femoral head between them. The two cuts can be parallel or convergent, depending on the geometry of the femoral head. When the femoral head is enlarged in line with the femoral neck (medial-lateral), the two cuts are parallel. When the femoral head is enlarged in both the AP and medial-lateral directions, it should be resected in a wedge shape with the base of the wedge anterolateral and the apex of the wedge posterior-medial. In the rare cases when the femoral head is enlarged in a proximal to distal direction together with AP direction, the wedge should be based superoanteriorly. Before making the osteotomy, the line of the osteotomy should be measured along the circumference of the femoral head. The length of this line should be the same for both osteotomies, thus ensuring that the lateral mobile segment of the femoral head will match the medial stable part of the femoral head. The osteotomy should also be parallel to the femoral neck. The lateral cut which is made first includes the superior part of the femoral neck to avoid damaging the retinacular vessels that provide circulation to this segment.[16,26] The medial part of the femoral head derives its blood supply from the posteromedial branch of the medial circumflex femoral artery, similar to a Pipkin II fracture.[16,26,27] Prior to the osteotomy, a posterior retinacular flap should be created to mobilize the vascular pedicles of the segments away from the back of the femur and the osteotomy line. The osteotomy is made with an oscillating saw. The author's preference is to use a saw with an oscillating tip because it cuts from its tip without the blade of the saw moving. The saw cut stops just short of the posterior cortex. A sharp, thin osteotome is used to crack the posterior cortex, thus avoiding injury to the vascular pedicles. After the first osteotomy, the lateral segment is free and can be mobilized on its vascular pedicle. The medial osteotomy is made in the same fashion. The segment of femoral head that is resected is removed, peeling off any remaining soft tissues posteriorly. Care should be taken not to narrow the femoral neck too much with the second cut. This goal can be achieved by taking a minimal amount of femoral neck with the first cut and by limiting the amount of neck resected with the second cut. After the osteotomies are completed, the lateral segment of femoral head should be advanced medially. The two should be fitted together as best as possible. If one is shorter anteroposteriorly from the other, the congruity of the osteotomy should be optimized posteriorly. The anterolateral part of the femoral head is normally outside of the acetabulum and only enters the joint with flexion and internal rotation or abduction. Furthermore, a negative cartilage defect is well tolerated whereas a positive step is harmful. Any gaps or defects can be filled with autogenous bone graft from the resected femoral head segment. The lateral segment can be stabilized with 4.5-mm cannulated headless screws. Three guide wires are inserted from the lateral to the medial fragment. Before drilling over these guide wires, the shape of the femoral head is measured again with the spherical templates. If it is not spherical, consider resecting more of the lateral segment. After measuring the length of the wire, the appropriate cannulated drill is used and the headless screw inserted. It is important to make sure that the screw does not protrude through the medial/inferior articular surface of the femoral head or from the lateral insertion site. Two screws are put through the femoral head articular surface laterally, and one screw is inserted across the femoral neck portion of the lateral segment. Because the femoral neck is narrowed and weakened by this resection, it is at risk of stress fracture. The author prefers to insert a prophylactic 4.5-mm solid screw up the femoral neck. A guide wire is drilled from the fovea to the lateral femur parallel to the femoral neck in the medial stable part of the femoral

head and neck. The wire can be overdrilled with a cannulated 3.2-mm drill from the lateral side. A 4.5-mm screw of the correct length is then inserted up the femoral neck from the lateral side. The length of this screw should not exit through the medial femoral head but should extend the entire length of the femoral head and neck. It is important to insert this screw before reducing the femoral head into the acetabulum. In one case the author reduced the hip into joint. The femoral head got stuck on the anterior lip of the acetabulum and the large lever arm force of the reduction maneuver was able to fracture the narrowed femoral neck. Test the movement of the femoral head in the acetabulum. There should be no impingement. The femoral head should be completely stable to flexion and extension because the anteroposterior shape of the large medial part of the femoral head has not been changed. There may be medial-lateral instability and inferior-superior instability, depending on the shape of the acetabulum and on the capsular laxity created by the reduced femoral head size. There is always medial-lateral laxity if there is proximal-distal instability. However, if there is a normally shaped acetabulum there can be medial-lateral instability without proximal-distal instability. Medial-lateral instability alone is caused by capsular laxity due to the redundant capsule following reduction of the intracapsular femoral head volume. This instability can usually be successfully stabilized by tightening the capsule. The femur should be slightly abducted with a bump placed between the two thighs. The posterior capsule, which is attached laterally, should be advanced medially by using supra-acetabular suture anchors. The anterior capsule should be advanced laterally and posteriorly by suturing to the posterior capsule and suture anchors into the anterolateral femur. Once the capsule is closed, the stability of the hip can be tested under image intensifier visualization. The other type of instability is caused by dysplasia of the acetabulum due to remodeling of the acetabulum. In these cases, when the femoral head is reduced a large space can be seen laterally between the articular surface of the acetabulum and the femoral head. In these cases one should consider a reshaping of the acetabulum. Because the entire lateral rim of the acetabulum is exposed and the inside of the acetabulum is visible, an incomplete osteotomy can be performed to hinge down the lateral wall of the acetabulum to better contain the femoral head and to be more congruous to the femoral head shape.[28] This method is equivalent to an adult version of the Dega osteotomy.[29] The osteotomy gap should be filled with a bone graft.[16] The resected part of the femoral head can be used for this, and if additional bone is required an allograft is used. These grafts are usually stable without internal fixation. The acetabular osteotomy is combined with the capsular tightening capsulorrhaphy described earlier. After the capsular repair, the greater trochanter can be reattached and advanced. The greater trochanter is almost always high in cases of Perthes. Furthermore, with coxa breva its moment arm is short. It should be advanced both laterally and distally, producing what is referred to as a relative neck lengthening. The greater trochanter is fixed with 3 identical-length 3.2-mm drill bits. Using the image intensifier, these are drilled from proximal lateral to distal medial. The length of these is measured using a free 3.2-mm drill bit and a ruler. Each drill bit is sequentially replaced with a 4.5-mm screw and a large fragment washer. These 3 screws and washers give excellent fixation of the greater trochanter. The rest of the closure includes the vastus lateralis, fascia lata over a drain, Scarpa's fascia, and subcutaneous and skin layers. Intraoperative radiographs should be taken to make sure that the femoral head is well reduced in the acetabulum. If the femoral head is laterally subluxed, consideration should be given to application of a temporary articulated spanning external fixator to reduce and hold the femoral head in place for 6 weeks while the capsule heals.

Postoperatively, the patient can be placed in continuous passive motion. The author prefers to use this modality at home for 6 weeks. This method should be combined with physical therapy to maintain the active and passive range of flexion and extension of the hip joint. Because continuous passive motion does not fully extend the hip, the therapist should make sure to stretch the hip to full extension. The hip may be passively abducted for the first 6 weeks. Active abduction should be avoided until the greater trochanter is healed (usually at 6 weeks). Passive and active adduction and external rotation range of motion should be avoided because they stress the capsular repair and the trochanteric fixation. These motions can be resumed after 6 weeks. Weight bearing is restricted to touch-down weight bearing for 3 months. After 6 weeks the extremes of motion should be stretched passively. To ensure that this is correctly done, the physical therapist should be educated about the use of the contralateral hip to lock the pelvis. For example, to maximize abduction stretch the contralateral hip should first be maximally abducted to lock the pelvis from moving as one stretches the affected hip into abduction. Full extension of the hip requires first flexing both hips, then leaving the contralateral

hip in maximum flexion (Thomas test) while pushing the affected hip into extension. Full flexion requires prior hyperextension of the contralateral hip before stretching the affected hip into flexion; this locks the pelvis into full extension so that all flexion motion seen is real. Finally, internal and external rotation can best be done by rotation of the contralateral hip into internal and external rotation, respectively.

RESULTS

The femoral head maximum diameter was an average of 133% larger than the opposite normal side on the AP view (range 115%–160%). Compared with itself, the femoral head after reduction was an average of 96% the diameter of the opposite normal side (range 91%–100%). Compared with the preoperative diameter, the femoral head was reduced by an average of 25% (range 13%–43%) (**Figs. 2** and **3**; see **Table 1**).

In all 20 patients the femoral head and greater trochanteric osteotomy was healed. The greater trochanter osteotomy was usually healed by 6 weeks and the FHRO was healed by 12 weeks. Five patients also underwent a pelvic osteotomy, all of which also healed uneventfully. Three of the pelvic osteotomies (Wagner 1 types)[28] were performed at the time of the index procedure as already described, while 2 had the Ganz periacetabular osteotomy performed 6 months after the index procedure.[30] A small arthrotomy at the time of the delayed pelvic osteotomy revealed a completely healed femoral head surface including the cartilage. Small drill holes lateral and medial to the osteotomy line revealed active bleeding in both of these cases.

In 5 patients an articulated external fixator was applied across the hip joint to help maintain the reduction of the femoral head in the acetabulum. Only 2 of these had the application performed at the index procedure. The other 3 had the external fixator applied 2 weeks after surgery when the first postoperative radiograph showed lateral subluxation. All the fixators were removed after 6 weeks, and recurrent subluxation did not occur. There was one AVN with fragmentation that occurred 18 months after the head reduction osteotomy. None of the other cases showed evidence of AVN. All but 2 patients in this study had follow-up longer than 18 months. This AVN patient was the only one in this series with an open femoral head physis at the time of the osteotomy, and the only one to have undergone a previous varus osteotomy, which altered and complicated the resection osteotomy. One year after the head reduction osteotomy, a valgus intertrochanteric osteotomy was performed. Finally, this case also

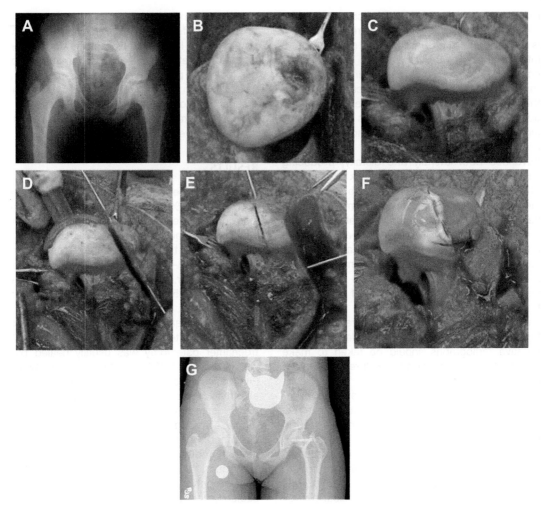

Fig. 2. An 11-year-old girl with femoral head deformity following Perthes disease, with onset at age 6 years. (*A*) Anteroposterior (AP) radiograph of the pelvis showing left coxa magna with saddle-shaped femoral head. (*B*) Superior view of the femoral head after surgical dislocation. (*C*) Lateral view of the femoral head after surgical dislocation, showing the saddle shape. (*D*) Lateral osteotomy. (*E*) Medial osteotomy. (*F*) Femoral head reduction. (*G*) AP radiograph of the pelvis 3 years after FHRO.

had the largest resection of the femoral head of any case (38%) and had the most preoperative subluxation and acetabular dysplasia of any case in the study. A periacetabular (Dega-like) osteotomy was performed at the time of the head reduction surgery and an external fixator was used postoperatively. The AVN case was also 1 of the 4 bilateral cases.

All patients who had good range of flexion-extension motion of the hip preoperatively had excellent full range of motion after healing. Eight patients with very stiff hip flexion-extension range of motion showed initial improvement, but 5 of these developed marked restricted range of motion by 1 year of follow-up. All 8 of these had advanced degeneration of the hip cartilage at the time of surgical dislocation. Five of the 8 are now painless.

Only 3 patients experienced pain during follow-up. Two have been treated by a hip replacement, while a repeat hip dislocation is planned on the other. Patients with normal range of motion, no pain, and no limp were classified as excellent. Those with improved range of motion from preoperatively but less than 80% of normal, no pain, and mild limp were classified as good. Patients with very stiff hips, moderate limp, but no pain were classified as fair. Patients with significant pain, stiffness, and limp were considered poor. There were 7 excellent, 7 good, 3 fair, and 3 poor final results.

DISCUSSION

The misshapen femoral head has been an unsolved problem in orthopedics leading to pain, limp,

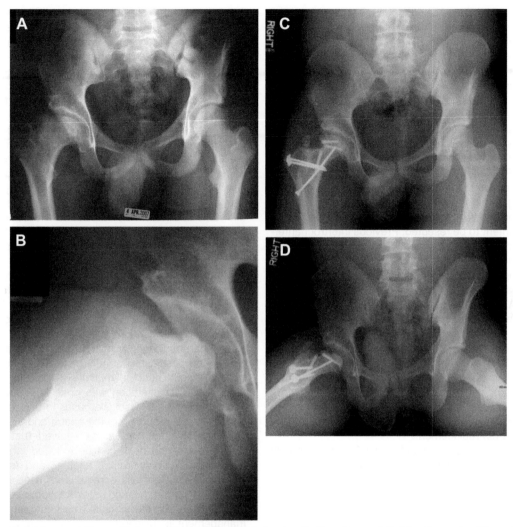

Fig. 3. A 14-year-old boy with femoral head deformity following Perthes disease. (*A*) AP radiograph of the pelvis showing coxa magna and saddle-shaped deformity. (*B*) Frog lateral radiograph showing coxa magna and deformity; this is a biplanar deformity. (*C*) AP radiograph of the pelvis 3 years following FHRO. The femoral head is well covered and is the same size at the opposite normal side. (*D*) Lateral pelvis radiograph after biplanar FHRO.

limitation of motion, impingement, acetabular dysplasia, and arthritis. In some cases valgus and valgus-extension osteotomy can alleviate many of the symptoms and can lead to hip preservation for 10 or more years.[8] Cheilectomy has been performed with variable results and without altering the natural history.[9–14] Most cases end up with some form of hip arthroplasty at a young age. Recent advances in the understanding, recognition, and treatment of femeroacetabular impingement have opened new opportunities, including safer more extensive cheilectomy techniques.[13,16,17,26] Most recently the Ganz safe surgical dislocation technique combined with a FHRO based on the femoral head vascular anatomy has for the first time offered the opportunity to restore sphericity to a nonspherical femoral head.[16,17]

The Stulberg and Mose classifications[21,23] classify and correlate femoral head sphericity to prognosis. Theoretically, if femoral head sphericity can be restored then the femoral head should last much longer. Because the longest follow-up in this study is 5 years, it is too early to comment on whether this procedure will alter the natural history. What can be said in this short-term follow-up is that by 18 months after surgery most patients have fully recovered their muscle strength and have no limp or pain, and avascular necrosis if present is already evident. Most patients have returned to unrestricted activities including sports and physical education. If a patient has good flexion-extension range of motion preoperatively, they maintain this and improve in all ranges of motion. If a patient has a lot of joint degeneration and restriction of flexion-extension range preoperatively, they often end up with permanent limitation of hip range of motion. Few patients ended up with residual pain. The 3 patients with poor results in this study all had residual pain. One developed avascular necrosis and the other 2 had preoperative stiffness and degenerative changes. The one case of avascular necrosis may be been predisposed because of 3 factors: open physis, large resection, and previous varus osteotomy.

Based on this study, the best indications for FHRO are misshapen femoral head, with good flexion and extension motion and limited cartilage degeneration on the acetabular side, and degeneration on the femoral side corresponding to the segment to be resected. Previous intertrochanteric osteotomy affects the ability to reduce the femoral head in the correct direction. The best shape to reduce is either an elliptical-shaped or a saddle-shaped femoral head.

Although the risk of avascular necrosis is significant, this study demonstrates that if the osteotomy is performed correctly this procedure can be accomplished with a very low rate of AVN. Most of these patients faced the prospect of an early hip replacement as one of the only alternative treatments. Therefore, the risk of AVN in a symptomatic patient may be acceptable because it does not burn any bridges with respect to performing a hip replacement.

Ganz's first report on the FHRO was in 2009. At that time he briefly reported the technique and the results of the first 11 patients: 9 for Perthes, 1 for AVN, and 1 for a high dislocation. The patients ranged in age from 9 to 15 years. In 3 hips postoperative instability was treated by a femoral varus osteotomy in 2 and a pariacetabular osteotomy (PAO) in 1 to stabilize the hip. Subsequently the next 3 cases were treated with PAO at the time of the FHRO.

In 2010 Ganz and colleagues reported on their first 14 FHROs since 2001. Eight hips also had a PAO at the same time as the index procedure while 3 had a PAO performed at a later date. In one case a varus intertrochanteric osteotomy was performed to treat subluxation, and in another a Colonna was performed at the same time. Therefore only 1 of their 14 cases did not have an additional procedure. None of the 14 cases developed avascular necrosis. No other details on this group were reported.

In a personal communication on one of their earliest and youngest patients, a recurrent femoral head deformity developed following a FHRO in a patient with an open proximal femoral physis. The two parts of the physis continued to grow in different directions, leading to a bifid femoral head. In the author's series the only case of AVN was in a child with an open femoral physis. A persistent open physis may therefore be a relative contraindication to this procedure.

This series of 20 FHRO osteotomies is currently the largest single-surgeon series of this procedure to the author's knowledge. It is also the first detailed study of FHRO. As in Ganz's series, the early results are very promising. This case series served to describe and report the short-term results of the technique. As noted previously, there are some modifications to the original technique. The surgical technique described is a more objective one, with intraoperative measurements of diameter and curvature to reduce the femoral head to as near normal as possible. This reduction in size is greater than that proposed by Ganz. However, as can be seen from the ratio of the postreduction to the size of the opposite normal side, reduction was achieved to within less than 10% of normal in all cases and to 100% of the normal diameter in 9 of the 16 unilateral cases. Although Ganz mentions that the segment resected can be triangular or trapezoidal in shape, there is no description of how to alter the shape of the femoral head in multiple planes. In this study, such an alteration was done in 5 cases. Furthermore, the 2 dysplasia cases in this series had a vertical reduction in the shape and size of the femoral head. This study showed that the femoral head and neck can be reduced in all 3 dimensions, namely frontal, sagittal, and transverse planes. Headless screws were used here instead of 3.5-mm headed screws recommended by Ganz. Finally, the surgical and postoperative management is outlined in much greater detail.

Longer term follow-up is important to determine whether the early excellent results will hold up, and whether the natural history of the disease will be altered by this osteotomy procedure.

REFERENCES

1. Grzegorzewski A, Synder M, Kozłowski P, et al. The role of the acetabulum in Perthes disease. J Pediatr Orthop 2006;26:316–21.
2. Kim HK, Randall TS, Bian H, et al. Ibandronate prevents femoral head deformity following ischemic necrosis of the capital femoral epiphysis in immature pigs. J Bone Joint Surg Am 2005;87:550–8.
3. Lopes N. Transepiphyseal head neck drilling for Perthes disease. Rev Portuguese Ortop Traum 1994;2(4):395–404.
4. Herring JA, Kim HT, Brown R. Legg-Calvé-Perthes disease, part II: prospective multicenter study of the effect of treatment on outcome. J Bone Joint Surg Am 2004;86:2121–34.

5. Beer Y, Smorgick Y, Oron A, et al. Long-term results of proximal femoral osteotomy in Legg-Calvé-Perthes disease. J Pediatr Orthop 2008;28(8):819–24.

6. Wenger DR, Pring ME, Hosalkar HS, et al. Advanced containment methods for Legg-Calvé-Perthes disease: results of triple pelvic osteotomy. J Pediatr Orthop 2010;30(8):749–57.

7. Segev E, Ezra E, Wientroub S, et al. Treatment of severe late onset Perthes' disease with soft tissue release and articulated hip distraction: early results. J Pediatr Orthop B 2004;13(3):158–65.

8. Clohisy JC, St John LC, Nunley RM, et al. Combined periacetabular and femoral osteotomies for severe hip deformities. Clin Orthop Relat Res 2009;467:2221–7.

9. Baksi DP. Palliative operations for painful old Perthes' disease. Int Orthop 1995;19:46–50.

10. Erard MC, Drvaric DM. Cheilectomy of the hip in children. J Surg Orthop Adv 2004;13:20–3.

11. Garceau GJ. Surgical treatment of coxa plana. J Bone Joint Surg Br 1964;46:779–80.

12. Rebello G, Spencer S, Millis MB, et al. Surgical dislocation in the management of pediatric and adolescent hip deformity. Clin Orthop Relat Res 2009;467:724–31.

13. Klisic P, Blazevic U, Seferovic O. Indication for treatment in coxa plana. Int Orthop 1997;1:33–5.

14. Shin SJ, Kwak HS, Cho TJ, et al. Application of ganz surgical hip dislocation approach in pediatric hip diseases. Clin Orthop Surg 2009;1(3):132–7.

15. Rowe SM, Jung ST, Cheon SY, et al. Outcome of cheilectomy in Legg-Calvé-Perthes disease. Minimum 25-year follow-up of five patients. J Pediatr Orthop 2006;26(2):204–10.

16. Ganz R, Huff TW, Leunig M. Extended retinacular soft tissue flap for intraarticular hip surgery: surgical technique, indications, and results of its application. Instr Course Lect 2009;58:241–55.

17. Ganz R, Horowitz K, Leunig M. Algorithm for combined femoral and periacetabular osteotomies in complex hip deformities. Clin Orthop Relat Res 2010;468(12):3168–80.

18. Sponseller PD, McBeath AA, Perpich M. Hip arthrodesis in young patients. A long-term follow-up study. J Bone Joint Surg Am 1984;66(6):853–9.

19. Rozbruch SR, Paley D, Bhave A, et al. Ilizarov hip reconstruction for the late sequelae of infantile hip infection. J Bone Joint Surg Am 2005;87(5):1007–18.

20. Boyd HS, Ulrich SD, Seyler TM, et al. Resurfacing for Perthes disease an alternative to standard hip arthroplasty. Clin Orthop Relat Res 2007;465:80–5.

21. Mose K. Methods of measuring in Legg-Calvé-Perthes disease with special regard to the prognosis. Clin Orthop 1980;150:103–9.

22. Rowe SM, Moon ES, Song EK, et al. The correlation between coxa magna and final outcome in Legg-Calvé-Perthes disease. J Pediatr Orthop 2005;25:22–7.

23. Stulberg SD, Cooperman DR, Wallensten R. The natural history of Legg-Calvé-Perthes disease. J Bone Joint Surg Am 1981;63:1095–108.

24. Leunig M, Beaulé PE, Ganz R. The concept of femoroacetabular impingement current status and future perspectives. Clin Orthop Relat Res 2009;467:616–22.

25. Ganz R, Gill T, Gautier E, et al. Surgical dislocation of the adult hip: a technique with full access to the femoral head and acetabulum without the risk of avascular necrosis. J Bone Joint Surg Br 2001;83:1119–24.

26. Gautier E, Ganz K, Krügel N, et al. Anatomy of the medial femoral circumflex artery and its surgical implications. J Bone Joint Surg Br 2000;82:679–83.

27. Sevitt S, Thompson RG. The distribution and anastomosis of the arteries supplying the head and neck of the femur. J Bone Joint Surg Br 1965;47:560–73. 22. 23.

28. Grudziak JS, Ward WT. Dega osteotomy for the treatment of congenital dysplasia of the hip. J Bone Joint Surg Am 2001;83(6):845–54.

29. Wagner H. Experiences with spherical acetabular osteotomy for the correction of the dysplastic acetabulum. Berlin: Springer-Verlag; 1978.

30. Ganz R, Klaue K, Vinh TS, et al. A new periacetabular osteotomy for the treatment of hip dysplasias. Technique and preliminary results. Clin Orthop Relat Res 1988;232:26–36.

Treatment of the Symptomatic Healed Perthes Hip

Eduardo N. Novais, MD[a], John Clohisy, MD[b],
Klaus Siebenrock, MD[c], David Podeszwa, MD[d],
Daniel Sucato, MD[d], Young-Jo Kim, MD, PhD[a,*]

KEYWORDS

- Legg-Calvé-Perthes disease • Hip arthritis
- Periacetabular osteotomy • Surgical hip dislocation

Legg-Calvé-Perthes disease (LCPD) is a pediatric form of osteonecrosis that ultimately heals but can cause femoral head and acetabular deformities. The deformities can be complex and may cause femoroacetabular impingement, hip instability, or combinations of both, and may ultimately lead to degenerative joint disease and early osteoarthritis (OA) of the hip. In the long-term follow-up of LCPD, osteoarthritis is reported to be a direct function of femoral head sphericity and congruence of the joint.[1–3]

The normal hip is a multiaxial, highly congruent ball-and-socket joint that requires inherent stability to protect and maintain long-lasting articular cartilage function.[4] In addition, it should provide ample and free range of motion required during everyday activities. Instability of the hip is usually a result of acetabular undercoverage, and results in labral tear and cartilage damage at the acetabular rim. Unlike in developmental dysplasia of the hip, in LCPD acetabular dysplasia is a result of secondary acetabular remodeling caused by the aspherical head. Femoroacetabular impingement (FAI) involves abnormal, repetitive contact between the anterior femoral head and/or head-neck junction against the anterior aspect of the acetabular rim, and has been linked to the onset of early osteoarthritis of the hip.[5–8] While in the unstable dysplastic hip the femoral head can subluxate out of the acetabulum, in FAI the femoral head remains well centered; however, free range of motion is limited.[9] In LCPD, the femoral head may heal in an aspherical shape and may cause both cam and pincer types of impingement. Instability and impingement usually are thought to be distinct pathomechanical entities. However, in LCPD a hip may be unstable in upright activities and yet still impinge in hip flexion due to the aspherical femoral head. FAI in LCPD is most often due to intra-articular impingement from the aspherical femoral head (cam FAI).[7,10,11] Nevertheless, it may also be secondary to acetabular overcoverage due to a retroverted acetabulum (pincer FAI).[12,13] In addition to the deformities caused by the disease process, prior surgical procedure to contain the collapsing head may cause impingement as well. Prior innominate osteotomy or shelf procedure may cause pincer-type impingement.[14] In addition, intra-articular impingement may be caused by functional retroversion of the proximal femur secondary to the retroverted position of the articulating femoral head or secondary to prior femoral osteotomy.[15]

In addition to the two aforementioned mechanical conditions (FAI and dysplasia), the patient

[a] Department of Orthopaedic Surgery, Children's Hospital Boston, 300 Longwood Avenue, Hunnewell 2, Boston, MA 02115, USA
[b] Department of Orthopaedic Surgery, Washington University School of Medicine, 660 South Euclid Avenue, St Louis, MO 63110, USA
[c] Department of Orthopaedic Surgery, University of Bern, Bern, Switzerland
[d] Texas Scottish Rite Hospital, 2222 Welborn Street, Dallas, TX 75219, USA
* Corresponding author.
E-mail address: Young-jo.Kim@childrens.harvard.edu

Orthop Clin N Am 42 (2011) 401–417
doi:10.1016/j.ocl.2011.05.003
0030-5898/11/$ – see front matter © 2011 Elsevier Inc. All rights reserved.

with a healed LCPD may present with pain due to abductor fatigue secondary to abductor lever insufficiency (high-riding greater trochanter) and limb length inequality (shorter ipsilateral limb). Osteochondritic lesions in the femoral head, although rare, may also be a source of pain and mechanical symptoms (locking, catching).[16,17] Therefore, an extensive preoperative evaluation of the proximal femur and acetabular morphology is recommended. The treatment strategy should address all the ongoing mechanical problems that affect each individual hip.

These consequences of residual LCPD deformities have been recognized in the past, and various treatment strategies have been used and reported on in the literature. Impingement of the enlarged femoral head on the lateral lip of the acetabulum, the so-called hinge abduction,[16] is a well-described phenomenon in LCPD. Historically, valgus-extension intertrochanteric osteotomy was indicated for the treatment of hinge abduction.[18] Valgus osteotomy has also been recommended to address residual deformities after the healing phase of LCPD. Myers and colleagues[19] reported on the results of valgus osteotomy in 15 patients who had completed reossification and remodeling of LCPD. There was significant improvement in pain and function measured by the Harris Hips Score after 2 years, and no subsequent alteration at final follow-up at 6.5 years.

Before a femoral osteotomy is performed, a radiograph with the leg adducted should demonstrate improvement of joint congruence, and the location and extension of femoral head deformity should be estimated. Yoo and colleagues[11] postulated that an abnormal hinge movement varies according to whether the impingement is lateral or anterior. These investigators identified some patients in whom major aspherical portion on the femoral head (the so-called bump) was located anteriorly. In this case the classic valgus-extension osteotomy may not be indicated, because the extension component will further add to the anterior impingement.

In saddle-shaped epiphysis, resection of the extruded anterolateral portion of the femoral head (cheilectomy) has been recommended in the past.[20–22] In 1964 Garceau[20] postulated that "in late Legg-Calvé-Perthes disease osteoarthritic changes resulted from incongruity of the femoral head which, because of bulging on the outer side, impinged on the acetabular lip. The degenerative changes could be reduced or delayed if the head of the femur was remolded. The operation should be done early, preferably before the age of twelve in boys and ten in girls, while remolding could still take place." Later, McKay[22] and Klisic[21] suggested that cheilectomy should not be performed at an early stage of the disease as had been previously recommended by Garceau.[20] Klisic[21] reported on cheilectomy in children aged 10 years or older. In children with severe subluxated epiphyses, cheilectomy resulted in 75% of ovoid femoral heads with no poor results. Among initially crushed epiphyses, acceptable results (ovoid and round femoral heads) were found after cheilectomy. Rowe and colleagues[23] reported on 5 patients with known poor prognosis who underwent partial head resection (cheilectomy) through an anterior approach. Cheilectomy was effective at reducing pain and improving range of hip motion during the early postoperative years; however, the clinical and radiographic results obtained at 25-year follow-up were not satisfactory. The investigators concluded that cheilectomy was ineffective at preventing the early osteoarthritic changes before age 40 years.

CONTEMPORARY APPROACH TO RESIDUAL LEGG-CALVÉ-PERTHES DEFORMITIES

In LCPD, resultant femoral head shape, growth disturbance of the proximal femoral physis, and secondary remodeling of the acetabulum can create complex deformities that may lead to abnormal mechanical function of the hip. With the advent of the safe surgical dislocation approach, clinicians now have an improved understanding of the pathoanatomy in LCPD. The intra-articular and extra-articular pathologies associated with healed LCPD can be classified in the following manner.

Proximal Femoral Pathoanatomy

Residual proximal femoral deformity can be identified as intra-articular, extra-articular, or in both locations. Intra-articular deformity can result from the aspherical femoral head, coxa magna, coxa plana, or a combination of these deformities, and can result in cam impingement, cam-induced impingement, or functional retroversion of the femoral head.

The cam impingement is a result of the aspherical femoral head entering a relatively spherical acetabulum.[8] The acetabulum cannot accommodate the large anterior segment of the femoral head. The anterior deformity can usually be identified on anteroposterior (AP) pelvic radiograph as the "sagging rope sign,"[24] a convex radiopaque line noted on AP plain radiographs of the proximal femur in patients with avascular necrosis of the femoral head. Repetitive injury from the cam impingement can lead to labral injury, progressing to labral avulsion from the acetabular rim, malacia of the acetabular cartilage, and eventual acetabular cartilage delamination.[6,8]

Cam-induced pincer impingement results from the coxa magna, coxa plana, or a combination of these deformities. The cam lesion (the large anterior femoral head) is too large to enter the joint, thus impinging on the acetabular rim.[8] The cam-induced pincer impingement results in a linear impact of the femoral head on the acetabular labrum causing primary labral injury and acetabular chondromalacia near the rim of the acetabulum.[6,8] Chronic pincer impingement can lead to labral ossification or a posterior-inferior contra coupe acetabular cartilage injury.[6]

Residual coxa magna may result in the articulating surface of the femoral head being out of line with the femoral neck. The femoral articular surface is frequently in the posteromedial superior portion of the femoral head, adjacent to an anterolateral inferior portion of the femoral head that protrudes from the acetabulum.[15] The anterolateral portion is considered the "false head" that is seen as a "sagging rope sign" and often blocks internal rotation of the hip. The posteromedial portion is considered the "true head" and is the remnant of the original articulating surface. This segment is retroverted relative to the anterolateral segment and results in a "functional retroversion" manifested clinically in an externally rotated gait.[15] The presence of the "false head" can also lead to cam-induced pincer impingement with the resultant labral and acetabular cartilage injury.

Greater trochanteric overgrowth is common in LCPD disease, and should be considered as an extra-articular pathoanatomy causing FAI. The combination of coxa breva (short and broad femoral neck) and high-riding trochanter can lead to anterior and/or posterior trochanteric impingement and represents a "functional coxa vara." Although the normal femoral neck-shaft angle is maintained, the level of the greater trochanter is cranial to the center of rotation of the femoral head. This situation manifests clinically as abductor weakness and a Trendelenburg limp, identical to that of a patient with true coxa vara.

Coxa breva can also create an abnormal relationship of the lesser trochanter relative to the ischium. Although rare relative to greater trochanteric overgrowth, enlargement of the lesser trochanter and/or decreased ischial-trochanteric distance can result in impingement of the lesser trochanter on the ischium. This impingement can result in pain, a snapping hip, decreased internal rotation of the hip, and/or decreased adduction of the hip.[25]

Acetabular Pathoanatomy

The acetabular dysmorphology that leads to altered hip biomechanics includes acetabular dysplasia, femoroacetabular incongruence, and acetabular retroversion.[12,13,26–28] The steep acetabular roof

that is the hallmark of acetabular dysplasia results in insufficient coverage of the femoral head and subsequent joint instability. The instability leads to increased shear stresses across the labrum, acetabular cartilage, and the compromised femoral head cartilage. Consequently, significant labral hypertrophy with or without intrasubstance labral injury and/or labral avulsion from the acetabular rim is frequently identified with associated cartilaginous injury at the acetabular rim.

A misshapen femoral head and acetabulum without true acetabular dysplasia can lead to femoroacetabular incongruity. The femoral head and acetabulum may be mismatched in shape, or the femoral head may be too large for a relatively shallow acetabulum. The incongruity leads to joint instability as a result of a complex motion pattern of femoral head translation and rotation within the acetabulum. Similar to acetabular dysplasia, incongruity and instability leads to increased shear stresses across the labrum and acetabular cartilage.[29]

Acetabular retroversion contributes to impaired hip range of motion and pincer impingement.[6,8] The cross-over sign[30] identified retroversion of the acetabulum on an AP pelvic radiograph in 31% to 42% of skeletally mature patients with residual deformity of healed LCPD disease.[12,13] A positive posterior wall sign, indicating a deficient posterior wall, was found in 21% of cases.[12]

All these deformities need to be recognized and their contribution to the patient's symptoms understood. In addition to the structural deformities, associated intra-articular abnormalities are common and contribute to patient symptoms, and should be addressed on a case-by-case basis; these include acetabular labral tears, articular chondral flaps and chondromalacia, osteochondral lesions, ligamentum teres ruptures, and loose bodies. These abnormalities contribute variably to patient symptoms and are to be addressed surgically on a case-by-case basis.

CLINICAL PRESENTATION AND IMAGING

Symptoms caused by mechanical abnormalities may develop in the residual phase of LCPD, and may cause hip pain in adolescents and young adults who were diagnosed and treated for LCPD as a child.[7] Typically the patient will present with groin pain that is aggravated by physical activities and sitting for long periods. Instability symptoms may present with groin pain after upright activities such as walking and running. Impingement symptoms are more common in positions of hip flexion and internal rotation. Early on, symptoms may be more characterized as stiffness and limitation of motion rather than pain. Mechanical symptoms of locking and catching may indicate the presence of intra-articular diseases including labral tears, chondral flaps, or an unstable osteochondral fragment.

Initial imaging should include an appropriate AP pelvic plain radiograph that can be obtained with the patient standing or supine. Quantitative measurements of acetabular coverage on the AP pelvis include the lateral center-edge angle of Wiberg[31] and the acetabular index of Tönnis.[32] The presence of a break in Shenton's line of greater than 5 mm characterizes joint subluxation and is a sign of mechanical instability of the hip. Acetabular retroversion can be identified by the presence of a cross-over sign[33] and the projection of the ischial spine into the pelvis.[34] The depth of the acetabulum can be evaluated using the ilioischial line as a reference: if the floor of the fossa acetabuli touches or is medial to the ilioischial line the hip is classified as coxa profunda, and if the medial aspect of the femoral head is medial to the ilioischial line it is classified as protrusio acetabuli.[35] In general, coxa profunda is rare in LCPD. Careful technique and analysis of the AP pelvis radiograph is important, as increased spinopelvic lordosis and pelvic rotation may falsely make the acetabulum appear retroverted.[36,37] In LCPD hip flexion contracture may be present, which may make the pelvis appear rotated or in a more lordotic position; therefore, interpretation of acetabular retroversion often needs to be interpreted with caution in LCPD. In addition to the pelvic radiograph, a false profile view of the acetabulum should be obtained to look for anterior undercoverage of the femoral head.[38]

A lateral view of the proximal femur (cross-table lateral,[39] frog-leg lateral,[40] or a Dunn view[41]) should also be obtained. The lateral view of the proximal femur adds information about the sphericity of the femoral head and the reduced head-neck offset. Quantitative evaluation of the head-neck junction includes measuring the alpha angle[42] and the head-neck offset ratio.[43] Functional radiographs, with or without an arthrogram, can provide additional information regarding the indication of a realignment femoral osteotomy in nonspherical hips.

Accurate measurement of acetabular and femoral version can be important information needed in the treatment planning of LCPD, and may require advanced imaging modalities such as computed tomography (CT) and magnetic resonance (MR) imaging. In LCPD, the anterolateral extrusion of the enlarged femoral head is believed to block internal rotation, while the posteromedial superior portion of the head that truly articulates in the acetabulum is retroverted and may functionally cause retroversion of the proximal femur.[15] CT scanning helps to quantify the femoral head-neck concavity and has

the advantage of 3-dimensional reconstruction, although it requires a dose of radiation.[44] MR arthrography with radial cuts rotating around the femoral neck axis allows assessment of the femoral head-neck junction shape and the labrum in its entire circumference.[45,46] Recently, delayed gadolinium-enhanced magnetic resonance imaging of cartilage has allowed direct assessment of cartilage matrix, and understanding of the complex damage pattern of hip joint cartilage and labrum after LCPD.[47]

SURGICAL TREATMENT TECHNIQUES
Periacetabular Osteotomy

Since its original description by Ganz and colleagues,[48] the Bernese periacetabular osteotomy (PAO) has gained popularity in the treatment of acetabular dysplasia.[49,50] The rationale and technique of PAO in patients with major aspherical femoral heads has been recently revised.[51,52] The goal is to mechanically stabilize the dysplastic hip, reducing acetabular rim loading to physiologic levels, and to avoid creating FAI. Clohisy and colleagues[52] recommended that a minimum of 95° of hip flexion should be present preoperatively as acetabular reorientation reduces hip flexion and abduction motion. The procedure is performed with the patient in the supine position. A modified Smith-Petersen anterior approach[53] is recommended to avoid extensive damage to the abductor musculature. Subperiosteal dissection of the inner table of the ilium is performed. Distally, the tensor fasciae latae compartment is entered and the sartorius identified. The lateral femoral cutaneous nerve within the sartorius fascia is therefore protected. The anterior-superior iliac spine (ASIS) is osteotomized or the sartorius is detached with a thin wafer of bone. With the leg in flexion and adduction, the reflected head of the rectus femoris is divided and the direct head of the rectus is elevated together with the iliocapsularis muscle from the hip capsule. The interval between the capsule and the iliopsoas tendon is developed and the osteotomy of the anterior portion of the ischium is performed. Osteotomy of the superior pubic ramus just medial to the iliopectineal eminence is then performed with a Gigli saw passed around the obturator foramen, with a microsagittal saw or with regular osteotomes. The supra-acetabular iliac osteotomy is performed with an oscillating saw aiming toward the apex of the sciatic notch and ending about 1 cm above the iliopectineal line. This corner will serve as the starting point of the posterior column osteotomy that is performed next. A Shanz screw is inserted into the acetabular fragment and is used to help mobilize the fragment into the corrected position.

Anatomically, the goal is to reorient the acetabular sourcil to nearly horizontal and restore the Shenton line, without lateralization of the hip center of rotation and no retroversion of the acetabulum (no cross-over or posterior wall sign). The acetabular fragment is then fixed with either 3.5- or 4.5-mm cortical screws. The osteotomy cuts, positioning, and fixation are monitored with intraoperative fluoroscopy. At this point an anterior arthrotomy is performed to inspect the acetabular labrum (and treat unstable labral tears) and to assess the femoral head-neck junction. In healed LCPD the large aspherical femoral head usually impinges against the acetabulum. An osteochondroplasty of the femoral head-neck junction is performed to optimize impingement-free range of motion. The capsule is closed and the rectus femoris and ASIS are repaired. The wound is closed in layers over a Hemovac drain.

Surgical Dislocation of the Hip

The surgical hip dislocation approach was initially described by Ganz and colleagues[54] after performing a dedicated study of the blood supply of the femoral head.[55] This approach allows complete access to the femoral head and acetabulum without risk of avascular necrosis of the femoral head.[54] The procedure is performed with the patient in the lateral decubitus position.[56,57] The entire lower extremity is prepped and draped, allowing visualization of the ASIS and the posterior superior iliac spine (PSIS), as they will serve as bony landmarks. A straight lateral incision (approximately 20 cm in length) is performed. In the past a Kocher-Langenbeck approach was used (splitting the muscle fibers of the gluteus maximus); however, nowadays a Gibson approach is preferred (the anterior muscle fibers of the gluteus maximus are freed from the fascia and the muscle is retracted posteriorly without splitting it). The fascia lata is split in line with the femoral shaft, exposing the vastus lateralis ridge and the posterior border of the gluteus medius. At this point the authors favor mobilizing the gluteus medius anteriorly and exposing the piriformis tendon. The interval between the piriformis tendon and the gluteus minimus is opened by sharp dissection. The inferior border of the gluteus minimus is dissected from underlying capsule. Performing this initial dissection will facilitate the exposure of the hip capsule further in the procedure. It is important to stay above (proximal to the superior border) the piriformis tendon to avoid injury to the anastomosis between the inferior gluteal artery and the medial femoral circumflex artery (MFCA).[55] Next, a 1- to 1.5-cm thick trochanteric osteotomy is performed with an oscillating saw, leaving the piriformis tendon and short external rotators intact on the base of the stable trochanter. The trochanteric piece is reflected and flipped anteriorly with the attached vastus lateralis and gluteus medius. The previously exposed capsular minimus is further elevated anteriorly off the hip capsule. The anterolateral portion of the vastus lateralis is released from the femur, with the hip in external rotation until the level of the gluteus maximus insertion. A capsulotomy is performed in a Z-shape fashion (right hip) or reverse Z-shape (left hip), with the longitudinal arm of the Z in line with the anterior femoral neck. The distal capsulotomy extends anterior proximally to the lesser trochanter while the proximal cut is performed along the acetabular rim until the piriformis tendon. With the capsule opened, the hip is carried through a range of motion with special attention to flexion and internal rotation. At this point, intra-articular and extra-articular causes of FAI can be dynamically determined. Flexion, adduction, and external rotation subluxates the hip, and the ligamentum teres is divided to allow complete dislocation of the femoral head. Three Hohman retractors are placed around the acetabulum, allowing complete exposure. The acetabulum articular cartilage and the labrum are inspected for the presence of labral and chondral lesions. The deformity of the femoral head (cam component) is accessed using spherical templates. Any nonspherical portion of the femoral head is removed with an osteotome and a burr. Reduction of the femoral head after osteochondroplasty should reveal improved flexion without impingement. If an osteochondroplasty is all that is required then the capsule is closed loosely and the trochanteric fragment is fixed with 2 or 3 3.5-mm cortical screws.

Development of Retinacular Soft-Tissue Flap: Relative Lengthening of the Femoral Neck and Femoral Head Reduction Osteotomy

In cases of healed LCPD the severity of the deformity (high-riding greater trochanter and short femoral neck) requires that osteochondroplasty of the femoral head-neck junction be performed in combination with a relative lengthening of the femoral neck (RLFN). The goals are to not only to improve abductor muscle function, but more importantly to correct the extra-articular source of impingement caused by the short femoral neck. Rarely, in extreme cases in patients between 10 and 15 years of age with no other surgical alternative, a resection of the middle portion of the persistently necrotic femoral head (femoral head reduction osteotomy [FHRO]) may be indicated in healed LCPD. The ideal indication is the patient who has restricted motion secondary to a large femoral head, whose peripheral cartilage is good but has a central segment of the head that has poor articular cartilage. In these situations an extended retinacular soft-tissue flap should be developed to protect the blood supply to the femoral head.[58]

To develop the retinacular flap, the femoral head should be reduced into the acetabulum.[58,59] The first step is to trim the posterosuperior portion of the stable greater trochanter down to the level of the femoral neck. The greater trochanter physis is identified. The portion of the greater trochanter proximal to the growth plate is mobilized with an osteotome, and the cancellous bone carefully removed from the periosteum. The periosteum is incised along the anterior neck beginning at the anterosuperior corner of the greater trochanter growth plate. The periosteum of the neck, including the retinaculum with the blood vessels and the external rotators, is gradually released. For RLFN the flap does not have to be developed in the whole circumference, as with FHRO. After the retinacular flap is developed the superior contour of the stable trochanteric segment is further trimmed in line with the femoral neck. The capsule is closed without tension. The mobile trochanter is advanced distally and fixed with 2 or 3 3.5-mm cortical screws.

Resection of the central portion of the femoral head (FHRO) is deemed possible because the extended retinacular flap preserves the blood supply to the superior portion of the femoral head. An additional branch of the medial circumflex femoral artery runs within the Weitbrecht ligament and supplies the inferior portion of the head.[60] The retinacular flap is extended posteriorly along the femoral neck while leaving it secured to the epiphysis. The lateral cut in the head/neck is made in line with the axis of the femoral neck, with a distal transverse cut made to allow mobilization. The medial cut is then made parallel to the first cut, and the segment is removed, allowing the remaining portions to be anatomically reduced. Two or 3 3.5-mm cortical screws are inserted from lateral/superior to medial/inferior.

Femoral Osteotomy

Valgus intertrochanteric osteotomy may be performed in isolation, but more often it is now performed in conjunction with a surgical dislocation approach to address intra-articular pathologies. Preoperative planning is mandatory to calculate the amount of valgization and the appropriate hardware to be used. In addition to valgus, flexion/extension and internal/external rotation may be added to the osteotomy. In LCPD the femoral head may be in a retroverted position, therefore a valgus/internal rotation osteotomy may be indicated.[61]

Greater Trochanter Advancement and True Femoral Neck Lengthening

Several different techniques have been reported for the transfer of the greater trochanter.[62–67] These methods include isolated transfer of the osteotomized fragment of the greater trochanter distally or a trochanteric transfer combined with a proximal femoral osteotomy. Wagner described the double osteotomy, using the base of the greater trochanter to lengthen the femoral neck and distally transferring the greater trochanter.[65] The Morscher double osteotomy[62,64,67] involves removing a segment of bone from the greater trochanteric base that is interposed between the trochanter and the femoral shaft. The distal osteotomy is at the subtrochanteric level and its angle corresponds with the desired neck-shaft angle. These osteotomies create several moving pieces, and internal fixation may be technically difficult. At present, relative neck lengthening is thought to be more effective than trochanteric transfer, due to the fact that in addition to the distal transfer, the extra-articular impingement around the large trochanteric base is visualized and surgically treated.

SURGICAL TREATMENT APPROACH

Successful treatment of LCPD patients with residual disease requires identification of individual deformities and associated soft-tissue abnormalities that contribute to the patient's symptoms. In this instance the most challenging aspect is to differentiate those patients with isolated FAI from patients with secondary acetabular dysplasia and instability and from those patients with both. In addition, it is important to understand the source of the conflict between the proximal femur and the acetabulum rim (femoral vs acetabular or combined; intra-articular vs extra-articular) to design the surgical plan.

The most common treatment options on the femoral side of the hip joint include intertrochanteric osteotomy,[68] relative neck lengthening,[58] true femoral neck lengthening,[62,64,65,67] trochanteric advancement,[63,66] and osteochondroplasty of the head/neck junction.[8] In extreme cases in patients between 10 and 15 years of age with limited surgical options, the femoral head reduction osteotomy has recently been performed.[59] On the acetabular side, extra-articular procedures include acetabular augmentation osteotomy[69,70] and redirectional osteotomies.[48] Complex deformities of both femur and acetabulum leading to instability and FAI usually require a combined approach.[52,71] Intra-articular procedures are common and include acetabular trimming with labral refixation,[56] labral repair, chondroplasty, microfracture, osteochondral fragment internal fixation, and osteochondral grafting.[72] The rather complex mismatch between the enlarged femoral head and the misshapen acetabulum limits the role for arthroscopic approach.[73,74]

The ultimate goal in the management of adolescents and young adults with FAI secondary to LCPD is to improve impingement-free range of motion and restore joint congruency. The recently described surgical dislocation of the hip allows full inspection of the joint and dynamic assessment of femoroacetabular contact during hip motion.[54] Through this approach of reshaping of the proximal femur via head-neck osteoplasty with or without a proximal femoral osteotomy, relative neck lengthening or trochanteric advancement, when indicated, can be performed.[59] In addition, it allows correction of focal anterosuperior acetabular overcoverage (pincer impingement) by an acetabular osteoplasty, and full access to the acetabular labrum and cartilage.[56]

Surgical management therefore should start with correction of the femoral deformity through a surgical dislocation approach. The authors carefully evaluate the causes of impingement preoperatively. If the enlarged femoral head with reduced head-neck offset is thought to be the isolated cause, an osteochondroplasty of the head-neck junction is performed. In these complex deformities the aspherical portion of the femoral head to be resected by the osteochondroplasty most often involves the epiphysis, and requires complete assessment of the femoral head-neck junction intraoperatively. Even though a labral tear may be present, it should not be treated without correction of the cam deformity. The indication to perform a relative neck-lengthening osteotomy after the osteochondroplasty is to correct extra-articular impingement due to a high-riding greater trochanter and a short wide neck. This situation is assessed after the femoral head-neck junction osteochondroplasty. If residual impingement of the neck and/or anterosuperior trochanteric bed is present in flexion/internal rotation then relative neck lengthening is performed. Trochanteric advancement is inherent to relative neck lengthening, and is advantageous in cases with trochanteric impingement and/or suboptimal abductor function due to the high trochanteric position. A general rule for advancement is that the trochanter should be positioned distally such that the tip of the trochanter is at the horizontal position of the femoral head center.

Table 1 Perthes femoral pathomorphology and treatment options	
Intra-Articular Impingement	
Cam	SHD + resection
Femoral head induced pincer	SHD + resection, ± head reduction, ± neck osteotomy
Functional retrotorsion	SHD, ± valgus/ flexion osteotomy
Extra-Articular Impingement	
Greater trochanter	SHD, ± relative neck lengthening
Lesser trochanter	SHD, ± distalization

Abbreviation: SHD, surgical dislocation of the hip.

When the osteoplasty and neck lengthening is not enough to correct the FAI, a femoral osteotomy is contemplated. The osteotomy should be performed at the intertrochanteric level, and the final decision on the type of osteotomy to be performed is based on preoperative evaluation of hip range of motion, functional radiographs, and radial sequence MR imaging. Finally, a perioperative assessment of the dynamic of the femoroacetabular contact during hip motion is done after the surgical dislocation of the hip. A flexion osteotomy is indicated when the anterolateral impingement area is too large to be completely removed. When the articulating portion of the femoral head is retroverted and functional retroversion of the proximal femur is present, a flexion-internal rotation osteotomy may be necessary to realign the lower extremity and reestablish a more functional arc of motion. Alternatively, a valgus-producing femoral osteotomy may be required if the patient has had a previous varus producing osteotomy with a major varus deformity and associated leg-length discrepancy. After correction of the femoral deformity it is crucial to evaluate the acetabulum, which may be dysplastic with undercoverage of the femoral head. Intraoperative

Table 2 Perthes acetabular pathomorphology and treatment options	
Acetabular Pathomorphology	
Acetabular dysplasia	PAO
Acetabular retrotorsion	Acetabular Rim Trimming; ± PAO
Joint incongruity	± Femoral Osteotomy; ± PAO

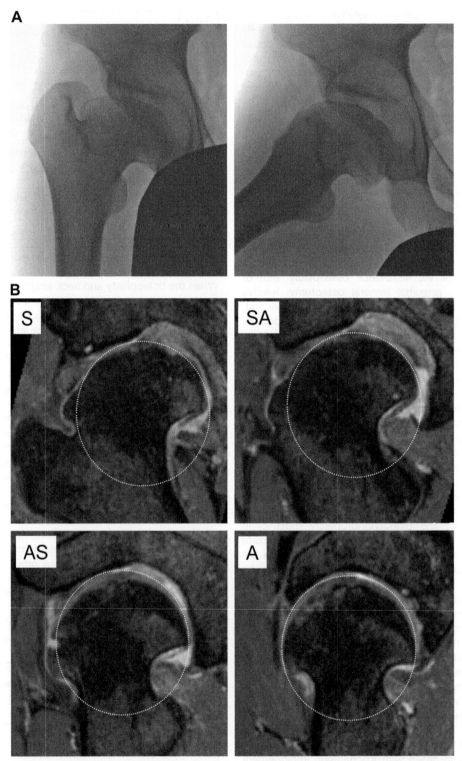

Fig. 1. Typical case of a 17-year-old with residual impingement due to LCPD. (*A*) Anteroposterior (AP) and lateral radiographs demonstrate the high-riding trochanter as well as the aspherical femoral head. (*B*) Radial MR image shows the aspherical femoral head in the superior (S) to anterior-superior (AS/SA) portion of the femoral head-neck junction. (*C*) AP and lateral radiographs following surgical dislocation and osteochondroplasty of the femur combined with a relative neck lengthening.

C

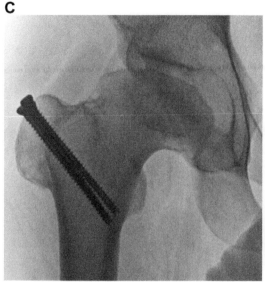 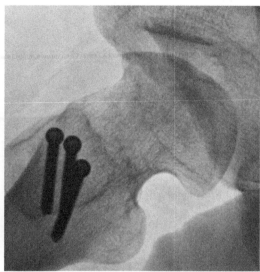

Fig. 1. (*continued*)

range-of-motion examination, fluoroscopic analysis with functional views, and direct visualization of hip stability are used to determine the need for additional stabilization of the joint. Anterior stability is checked with extension/external rotation while lateral and posterosuperior stability are assessed during a functional flexion/extension range-of-motion test. In this situation symptoms related to mechanical instability may persist and may be improved by a redirectional periacetabular osteotomy; this is done by repositioning the patient and performing a second anterior approach. In some patients with previous shelf augmentation of the acetabulum and pincer-type impingement, the overcoverage may be corrected by an osteoplasty of the acetabular rim with labrum refixation. Acetabular reorientation in LCPD should be performed with heightened attention to creating secondary FAI. Commonly the acetabular reorientation is "conservative" in order to avoid this potential problem. The authors' preliminary results on 15 patients who underwent a surgical dislocation of the hip for the management of FAI secondary to LCPD revealed that the WOMAC scores were reduced from a preoperative score of 9.6 to 5.1 postoperatively.[75]

Residual deformities from LCPD are complex and may produce intra-articular FAI, extra-articular FAI, structural instability (secondary acetabular dysplasia), and associated intra-articular abnormalities (labral tears, chondral flaps, osteochondral lesions, and chondromalacia). The authors believe that following careful preoperative

planning including accurate measurement of hip range of motion, radiographs (AP pelvis, false profile, and lateral hip) associated with MR imaging (radial sequences), a surgical dislocation of the hip allows a safe approach to correct the femoral and acetabular deformities responsible for FAI secondary to LCPD in adolescents. Associated hip instability is not uncommon, and correction with acetabular reorientation may be required. The possible surgical procedures necessary for the femoral and acetabular deformities are summarized in **Tables 1** and **2**.

CASE EXAMPLES

The majority of cases of impingement due to LCPD will require a femoral head-neck junction osteochondroplasty to relieve intra-articular impingement as well as a relative neck lengthening to relieve extra-articular impingement. **Fig. 1**A, B illustrates a typical case of a 17-year-old with residual impingement due to LCPD. Panel A illustrates the high-riding trochanter as well as the aspherical femoral head. The radial MR image shown in panel B shows the aspherical femoral head in the superior to anterior-superior portion of the femoral head-neck junction. Through a surgical dislocation approach, both an osteochondroplasty of the femur and a relative neck lengthening was performed (**Fig. 1**C). This procedure relieves pain by decreasing impingement in the joint and improves motion by relieving extra-articular impingement.

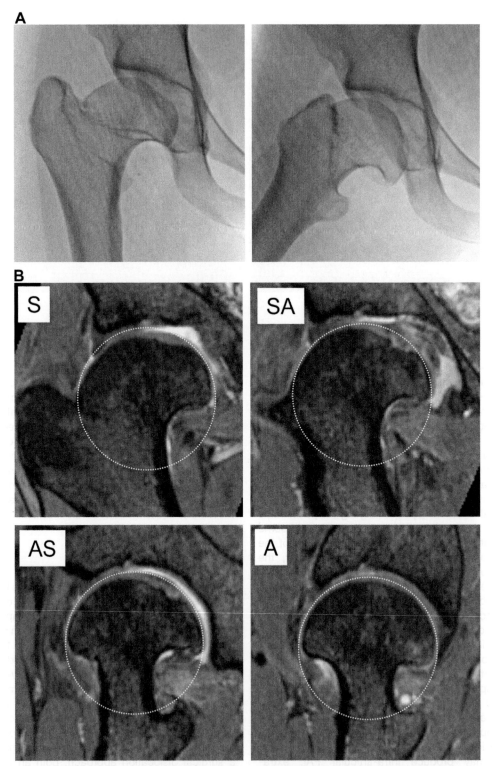

Fig. 2. Case of an 18-year-old girl with hip pain due to healed LCPD. (*A*) Preoperative radiographs show a high-riding greater trochanter and slightly aspherical femoral head. (*B*) Radial MR image demonstrates that the femoral head itself is relatively spherical. (*C*) Postoperative radiographs following relative neck lengthening because most of the impingement was extra-articular in nature.

C

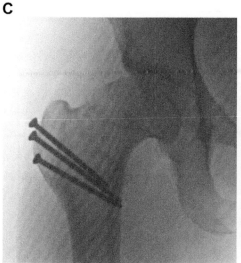 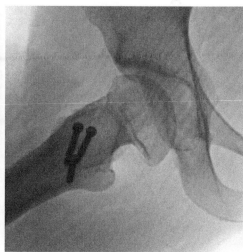

Fig. 2. (*continued*)

In the case of an 18-year-old woman with hip pain due to healed LCPD, the preoperative radiographs show a high-riding trochanter and slightly aspherical femoral head (**Fig. 2**A). Close inspection of the radial MR image shows (**Fig. 2**B) that the femoral head itself is relatively spherical. Most of the impingement was extra-articular in nature, which was treated with a relative neck lengthening (**Fig. 2**C).

In cases of LCPD with a large extruded femoral head, function retroversion may be present, whereby the articulating femoral head is in the posterior-medial position. An 11-year-old boy with partially healed LCPD shows a large anteriorly extruded femoral head (**Fig. 3**A). Axial CT sections demonstrate the retroverted position of the articulating femoral head (**Fig. 3**B). To fully correct the deformity, a large osteochondroplasty was performed as well as a flexion, derotation intertrochanteric osteotomy (**Fig. 3**C).

Often an aspherical femoral head will remodel the acetabulum to fit the femoral head, which may result in a dysplastic acetabulum, as seen in a 15-year-old patient (**Fig. 4**A). At present, there is no clear measure of hip instability in LCPD. In this case a femoral osteochondroplasty and a relative neck lengthening were performed, but the patient remained symptomatic with upright activities. These symptoms resolved once the hip was stabilized with a periacetabular osteotomy (**Fig. 4**B).

In rare instances the lesser trochanter may cause impingement as well. In the case of a 15-year-old girl who developed avascular necrosis of the hip after open surgical reduction of a congenitally dislocated femoral head due to developmental dysplasia of the hip, the short femoral neck caused impingement of both the greater and lesser trochanters (**Fig. 5**A). Before corrective surgery, she presented with a shortening of the left lower limb of 5 cm, inguinal and lateral pain on ambulation, hip flexion of 80°, and only a minor capacity for hip rotation. Following the corrective surgery (relative lengthening of neck, distalization of the greater and lesser trochanter), the patient presented only with mild groin pain on prolonged walking, with flexion/extension of 90°/0° and internal/external rotation of 30°/20° (**Fig. 5**B).

Patients often have a large femoral head with the worst articular cartilage located in the central aspect of the femoral head, and have good articular cartilage on the peripheral aspects. When the principal complaint is restricted motion and pain at only the extremes of motion, then a central femoral head resection to remove the bad articular cartilage, to decrease the size of the femoral head, and to improve motion is performed. This action requires a very careful surgical technique to create the retinacular flap and preserve the blood flow to the femoral head. A 15-year-old woman complained primarily of a restricted range of motion in rotation with (internal rotation of 0° and external rotation of 20°) and flexion (limited to 80°) without significant pain within the range. The radiographs (**Fig. 6**A) demonstrated a large femoral head with

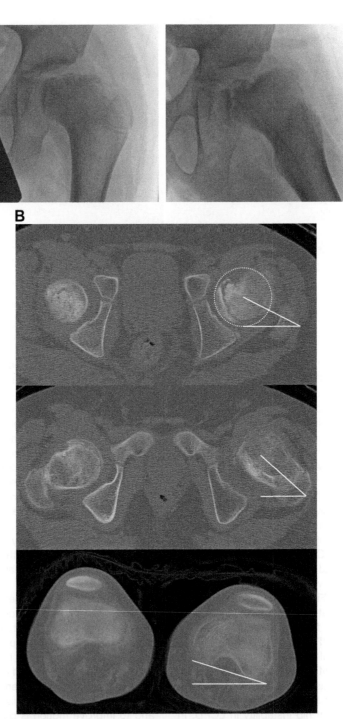

Fig. 3. A large extruded femoral head can lead to functional retroversion, due to the posterior-medial position of the articulating femoral head. (*A*) Radiographs of an 11-year-old boy with a partially healed LCPD demonstrating a large anteriorly extruded femoral head. (*B*) Axial CT scan sections demonstrate the retroverted position of the articulating femoral head. (*C*) Radiographs following osteochondroplasty combined with flexion, derotation, and intertrochanteric osteotomy.

C

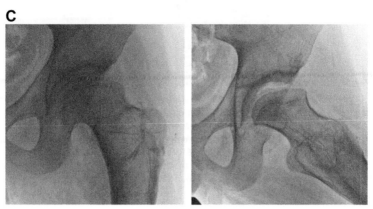

Fig. 3. (*continued*)

A

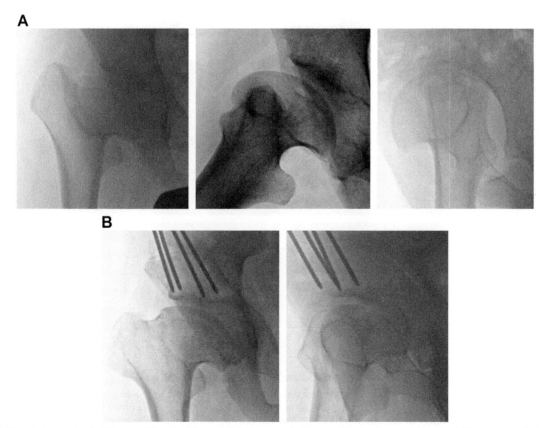

B

Fig. 4. An aspherical femoral head will remodel the acetabulum to fit the femoral head, which may result in a dysplastic acetabulum. (*A*) Radiographs of a 15-year-old boy. At present there is no clear measure of hip instability in LCPD. (*B*) Radiographs following a femoral osteochondroplasty with a relative neck lengthening and hip stabilization, with a periactabular osteotomy.

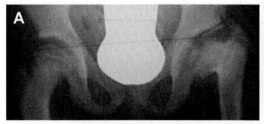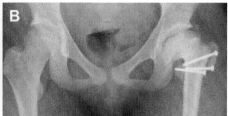

Fig. 5. Case of a 15-year-old girl who developed avascular necrosis of the hip after open surgical reduction of a congenitally dislocated femoral head due to developmental dysplasia of the hip. (*A*) Radiograph demonstrates a short femoral neck with impingement of both the greater and lesser trochanters. Before corrective surgery, she presented with a shortening of the left lower limb of 5 cm, inguinal and lateral pain on ambulation, hip flexion of 80°, and only a minor capacity for hip rotation. (*B*) Postoperative radiograph demonstrates relative neck lengthening with distalization of the greater and lesser trochanters. Following the corrective surgery the patient presented only with mild groin pain on prolonged walking, with flexion/extension 90°/0° and internal/external rotation of 30°/20°.

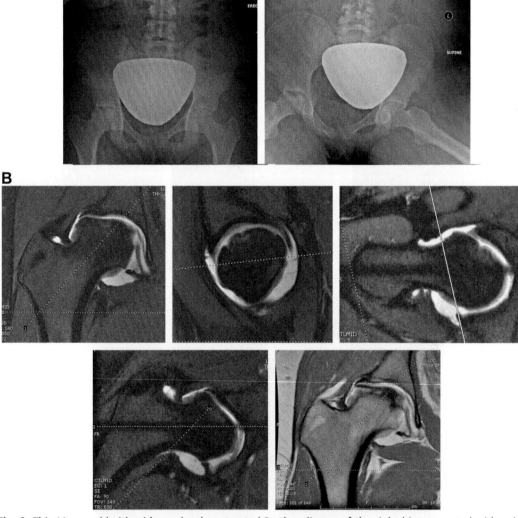

Fig. 6. This 14-year-old girl, with previously untreated Perthes disease of the right hip, presented with painful symptoms at the extremes of hip motion. (*A*) The AP and frog-leg lateral radiograph of the right hip demonstrate a depressed central aspect of the femoral head. (*B*) The MR arthrogram demonstrates reasonably good articular cartilage on the medial and lateral aspect of the femoral head, with a central osteochondral defect and a labrum that is elevated by the large lateral femoral head segment. (*C*) Intraoperative photograph demonstrating the central aspect of the femoral head being removed. The medial column of the femoral head has a pressure monitor in place to confirm good blood flow. (*D*) AP view of the right hip 2 years following surgery, demonstrating a healed proximal femur with resultant nearly-round femoral head that is congruent with the acetabulum.

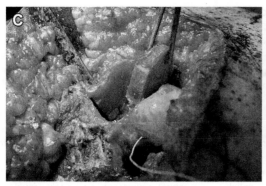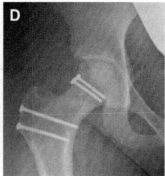

Fig. 6. (*continued*)

a central necrotic segment, confirmed by MR arthrogram, which also demonstrates some labral proximal migration secondary to the large anterior and lateral femoral head (**Fig. 6**B). In this case, a central femoral head resection (**Fig. 6**C) preserves the best articular cartilage and improves her range of motion significantly because a more normal-sized femoral head is now present (**Fig. 6**D).

REFERENCES

1. Mose K, Hjorth L, Ulfeldt M, et al. Legg Calvé Perthes disease. The late occurrence of coxarthrosis. Acta Orthop Scand Suppl 1977;169:1–39.

2. Stulberg SD, Cooperman DR, Wallensten R. The natural history of Legg-Calvé-Perthes disease. J Bone Joint Surg Am 1981;63(7):1095–108.

3. Weinstein SL. Legg-Calvé-Perthes disease: results of long-term follow-up. Hip 1985;28–37.

4. Bombelli R, Santore RF, Poss R. Mechanics of the normal and osteoarthritic hip. A new perspective. Clin Orthop Relat Res 1984;(182):69–78.

5. Beaule PE, Allen DJ, Clohisy JC, et al. The young adult with hip impingement: deciding on the optimal intervention. Instr Course Lect 2009;58:213–22.

6. Beck M, Kalhor M, Leunig M, et al. Hip morphology influences the pattern of damage to the acetabular cartilage: femoroacetabular impingement as a cause of early osteoarthritis of the hip. J Bone Joint Surg Br 2005;87(7):1012–8.

7. Eijer H, Podeszwa DA, Ganz R, et al. Evaluation and treatment of young adults with femoro-acetabular impingement secondary to Perthes' disease. Hip Int 2006;16(4):273–80.

8. Ganz R, Parvizi J, Beck M, et al. Femoroacetabular impingement: a cause for osteoarthritis of the hip. Clin Orthop Relat Res 2003;(417):112–20.

9. Leunig M, Beaule PE, Ganz R. The concept of femoroacetabular impingement: current status and future perspectives. Clin Orthop Relat Res 2009; 467(3):616–22.

10. Snow SW, Keret D, Scarangella S, et al. Anterior impingement of the femoral head: a late phenomenon of Legg-Calvé-Perthes' disease. J Pediatr Orthop 1993;13(3):286–9.

11. Yoo WJ, Choi IH, Chung CY, et al. Valgus femoral osteotomy for hinge abduction in Perthes' disease. Decision-making and outcomes. J Bone Joint Surg Br 2004;86(5):726–30.

12. Ezoe M, Naito M, Inoue T. The prevalence of acetabular retroversion among various disorders of the hip. J Bone Joint Surg Am 2006;88(2):372–9.

13. Sankar WN, Flynn JM. The development of acetabular retroversion in children with Legg-Calvé-Perthes disease. J Pediatr Orthop 2008;28(4):440–3.

14. Dora C, Mascard E, Mladenov K, et al. Retroversion of the acetabular dome after Salter and triple pelvic osteotomy for congenital dislocation of the hip. J Pediatr Orthop B 2002;11(1):34–40.

15. Kim HT, Wenger DR. "Functional retroversion" of the femoral head in Legg-Calvé-Perthes disease and epiphyseal dysplasia: analysis of head-neck deformity and its effect on limb position using three-dimensional computed tomography. J Pediatr Orthop 1997;17(2):240–6.

16. Grossbard GD. Hip pain during adolescence after Perthes' disease. J Bone Joint Surg Br 1981;63B(4): 572–4.

17. Kamhi E, MacEwen GD. Osteochondritis dissecans in Legg-Calvé-Perthes disease. J Bone Joint Surg Am 1975;57(4):506–9.

18. Quain S, Catterall A. Hinge abduction of the hip. Diagnosis and treatment. J Bone Joint Surg Br 1986; 68(1):61–4.

19. Myers GJ, Mathur K, O'Hara J. Valgus osteotomy: a solution for late presentation of hinge abduction in Legg-Calvé-Perthes disease. J Pediatr Orthop 2008; 28(2):169–72.

20. Garceau G. Surgical treatment of coxa plana. J Bone Joint Surg Br 1964;46:779–80.

21. Klisic PJ. Treatment of Perthes' disease in older children. J Bone Joint Surg Br 1983;65(4):419–27.

22. McKay DW. Cheilectomy of the hip. Orthop Clin North Am 1980;11(1):141–60.

23. Rowe SM, Jung ST, Cheon SY, et al. Outcome of cheilectomy in Legg-Calvé-Perthes disease: minimum 25-year follow-up of five patients. J Pediatr Orthop 2006;26(2):204–10.

24. Apley AG, Wientroub S. The sagging rope sign in Perthes' disease and allied disorders. J Bone Joint Surg Br 1981;63(1):43–7.

25. Patti JW, Ouellette H, Bredella MA, et al. Impingement of lesser trochanter on ischium as a potential cause for hip pain. Skeletal Radiol 2008;37(10): 939–41.

26. Bellyei A, Mike G. Acetabular development in Legg-Calvé-Perthes disease. Orthopedics 1988;11(3): 407–11.

27. Eijer H. Towards a better understanding of the aetiology of Legg-Calvé-Perthes' disease: acetabular retroversion may cause abnormal loading of dorsal femoral head-neck junction with restricted blood supply to the femoral epiphysis. Med Hypotheses 2007;68(5):995–7.

28. Kamegaya M, Shinada Y, Moriya H, et al. Acetabular remodelling in Perthes' disease after primary healing. J Pediatr Orthop 1992;12(3):308–14.

29. Klaue K, Durnin CW, Ganz R. The acetabular rim syndrome. A clinical presentation of dysplasia of the hip. J Bone Joint Surg Br 1991;73(3):423–9.

30. Reynolds D, Lucas J, Klaue K. Retroversion of the acetabulum. A cause of hip pain. J Bone Joint Surg Br 1999;81(2):281–8.

31. Wiberg G. Studies on dysplastic acetabula and congenital subluxation of the hip joint. With special reference to the complication of osteoarthritis. Acta Chir Scand 1939;83(Suppl 58):28–38.

32. Tonnis D. Normal values of the hip joint for the evaluation of X-rays in children and adults. Clin Orthop Relat Res 1976;(119):39–47.

33. Jamali AA, Mladenov K, Meyer DC, et al. Anteroposterior pelvic radiographs to assess acetabular retroversion: high validity of the "cross-over-sign". J Orthop Res 2007;25(6):758–65.

34. Kalberer F, Sierra RJ, Madan SS, et al. Ischial spine projection into the pelvis: a new sign for acetabular retroversion. Clin Orthop Relat Res 2008;466(3): 677–83.

35. Clohisy JC, Carlisle JC, Beaule PE, et al. A systematic approach to the plain radiographic evaluation of the young adult hip. J Bone Joint Surg Am 2008; 90(Suppl 4):47–66.

36. Clohisy JC, Carlisle JC, Trousdale R, et al. Radiographic evaluation of the hip has limited reliability. Clin Orthop Relat Res 2009;467(3):666–75.

37. Tannast M, Zheng G, Anderegg C, et al. Tilt and rotation correction of acetabular version on pelvic radiographs. Clin Orthop Relat Res 2005;438: 182–90.

38. Lequesne M, de Sèze S. [Le faux profil du bassin: nouvelle incidence radiographique pour l'etude de la hanche. Son utilité dans les dysplasies et les diferentes coxopathies]. Rev Rhum Mal Osteoartic 1961;28:643–52 [in French].

39. Eijer H, Leunig M, Mahomed M, et al. Cross-table lateral radiograph for screening of anterior femoral head-neck offset in patients with femoroacetabular impingement. Hip Int 2001;11:37–41.

40. Clohisy JC, Nunley RM, Otto RJ, et al. The frog-leg lateral radiograph accurately visualized hip cam impingement abnormalities. Clin Orthop Relat Res 2007;462:115–21.

41. Dunn DM. Anteversion of the nook of the femur; a method of measurement. J Bone Joint Surg Br 1952;34(2):181–6.

42. Barton C, Salineros MJ, Rakhra KS, et al. Validity of the alpha angle measurement on plain radiographs in the evaluation of cam-type femoroacetabular impingement. Clin Orthop Relat Res 2011;469(2): 464–9.

43. Peelle MW, Della Rocca GJ, Maloney WJ, et al. Acetabular and femoral radiographic abnormalities associated with labral tears. Clin Orthop Relat Res 2005;441:327–33.

44. Beaule PE, Zaragoza E, Motamedi K, et al. Three-dimensional computed tomography of the hip in the assessment of femoroacetabular impingement. J Orthop Res 2005;23(6):1286–92.

45. Horii M, Kubo T, Hirasawa Y. Radial MRI of the hip with moderate osteoarthritis. J Bone Joint Surg Br 2000;82(3):364–8.

46. Locher S, Werlen S, Leunig M, et al. MR-Arthrography with radial sequences for visualization of early hip pathology not visible on plain radiographs. Z Orthop Ihre Grenzgeb 2002;140(1):52–7 [in German].

47. Zilkens C, Holstein A, Bittersohl B, et al. Delayed gadolinium-enhanced magnetic resonance imaging of cartilage in the long-term follow-up after Perthes disease. J Pediatr Orthop 2010;30(2):147–53.

48. Ganz R, Klaue K, Vinh TS, et al. A new periacetabular osteotomy for the treatment of hip dysplasias. Technique and preliminary results. Clin Orthop Relat Res 1988;(232):26–36.

49. Clohisy JC, Barrett SE, Gordon JE, et al. Periacetabular osteotomy for the treatment of severe acetabular dysplasia. J Bone Joint Surg Am 2005;87(2): 254–9.

50. Matheney T, Kim YJ, Zurakowski D, et al. Intermediate to long-term results following the Bernese periacetabular osteotomy and predictors of clinical outcome. J Bone Joint Surg Am 2009;91(9):2113–23.

51. Beck M, Mast JW. The periacetabular osteotomy in Legg-Perthes-like deformities. Semin Arthroplasty 1997;(8):102–7.

52. Clohisy JC, Nunley RM, Curry MC, et al. Periacetabular osteotomy for the treatment of acetabular dysplasia associated with major aspherical femoral head deformities. J Bone Joint Surg Am 2007; 89(7):1417–23.

53. Murphy SB, Millis MB. Periacetabular osteotomy without abductor dissection using direct anterior exposure. Clin Orthop Relat Res 1999;(364):92–8.

54. Ganz R, Gill TJ, Gautier E, et al. Surgical dislocation of the adult hip a technique with full access to the femoral head and acetabulum without the risk of avascular necrosis. J Bone Joint Surg Br 2001; 83(8):1119–24.

55. Gautier E, Ganz K, Krugel N, et al. Anatomy of the medial femoral circumflex artery and its surgical implications. J Bone Joint Surg Br 2000;82(5):679–83.

56. Espinosa N, Beck M, Rothenfluh DA, et al. Treatment of femoro-acetabular impingement: preliminary results of labral refixation. Surgical technique. J Bone Joint Surg Am 2007;89(Suppl 2 Pt.1):36–53.

57. Spencer S, Millis MB, Kim YJ. Early results of treatment of hip impingement syndrome in slipped capital femoral epiphysis and pistol grip deformity of the femoral head-neck junction using the surgical dislocation technique. J Pediatr Orthop 2006;26(3):281–5.

58. Ganz R, Huff TW, Leunig M. Extended retinacular soft-tissue flap for intra-articular hip surgery: surgical technique, indications, and results of application. Instr Course Lect 2009;58:241–55.

59. Ganz R, Horowitz K, Leunig M. Algorithm for femoral and periacetabular osteotomies in complex hip deformities. Clin Orthop Relat Res 2010;468(12):3168–80.

60. Kalhor M, Beck M, Huff TW, et al. Capsular and pericapsular contributions to acetabular and femoral head perfusion. J Bone Joint Surg Am 2009;91(2):409–18.

61. Kim HT, Wenger DR. Surgical correction of "functional retroversion" and "functional coxa vara" in late Legg-Calvé-Perthes disease and epiphyseal dysplasia: correction of deformity defined by new imaging modalities. J Pediatr Orthop 1997;17(2):247–54.

62. Hasler CC, Morscher EW. Femoral neck lengthening osteotomy after growth disturbance of the proximal femur. J Pediatr Orthop B 1999;8(4):271–5.

63. Macnicol MF, Makris D. Distal transfer of the greater trochanter. J Bone Joint Surg Br 1991;73(5):838–41.

64. Buess P, Morscher E. Osteotomy to lengthen the femur neck with distal adjustment of the trochanter major in coxa vara after hip dislocation. Orthopade 1988;17(6):485–90 [in German].

65. Wagner H. Femoral osteotomies for congenital hip dislocation. In: Weil UH, editor. Progress in orthopedic surgery: acetabular dysplasia and skeletal dysplasia in childhood, vol. 2. New York: Springer-Verlag; 1978. p. 85.

66. Lascombes P, Prevot J, Allouche A, et al. Lengthening osteotomy of the femoral neck with transposition of the greater trochanter in acquired coxa vara. Rev Chir Orthop Reparatrice Appar Mot 1985;71(8): 599–601 [in French].

67. Hefti F, Morscher E. The femoral neck lengthening osteotomy. Orthoped Traumatol 1993;2(3):144–51.

68. Millis MB, Murphy SB, Poss R. Osteotomies about the hip for the prevention and treatment of osteoarthrosis. Instr Course Lect 1996;45:209–26.

69. Chiari K. Medial displacement osteotomy of the pelvis. Clin Orthop Relat Res 1974;(98):55–71.

70. Bennett JT, Mazurek RT, Cash JD. Chiari's osteotomy in the treatment of Perthes' disease. J Bone Joint Surg Br 1991;73(2):225–8.

71. Millis MB, Kim YJ. Rationale of osteotomy and related procedures for hip preservation: a review. Clin Orthop Relat Res 2002;(405):108–21.

72. Anderson LA, Erickson JA, Severson EP, et al. Sequelae of Perthes disease: treatment with surgical hip dislocation and relative femoral neck lengthening. J Pediatr Orthop 2010;30(8):758–66.

73. Kocher MS, Kim YJ, Millis MB, et al. Hip arthroscopy in children and adolescents. J Pediatr Orthop 2005; 25(5):680–6.

74. Roy DR. Arthroscopic findings of the hip in new onset hip pain in adolescents with previous Legg-Calvé-Perthes disease. J Pediatr Orthop B 2005;14(3):151–5.

75. Rebello G, Spencer S, Millis MB, et al. Surgical dislocation in the management of pediatric and adolescent hip deformity. Clin Orthop Relat Res 2009; 467(3):724–31.

Review of Total Hip Resurfacing and Total Hip Arthroplasty in Young Patients Who Had Legg-Calvé-Perthes Disease

Christopher R. Costa, MD, Aaron J. Johnson, MD,
Qais Naziri, MD, Michael A. Mont, MD*

KEYWORDS

• Perthes • THA • Total hip resurfacing • Young adult

Patients with Legg-Calvé-Perthes disease can often be successfully treated with femoral head–preserving measures, such as bracing, or containment procedures with osteotomies. However, in some cases, after resolution of the disease, the femoral head may proceed to collapse or progress to severe arthritis at a young age. If nonoperative methods have failed, the only treatment options available for these adolescents or young adults may be a total hip resurfacing or a total hip arthroplasty (THA). A study of the Danish registry of 135 patients (156 hips) treated for Legg-Calvé-Perthes disease found that 13% of patients required a THA procedure as opposed to none in an age-matched cohort of healthy patients after a mean follow-up of 47 years (range, 37–58 years).[1] This article focuses on the results and unique technical considerations of resurfacing and THA for patients who have severe hip osteoarthritis after resolved Legg-Calvé-Perthes disease.

TOTAL HIP RESURFACING

Because of younger age and higher activity levels seen in patients who have severe hip osteoarthritis after resolved Legg-Calvé-Perthes disease, total hip resurfacing may provide a more attractive alternative to conventional THA. Resurfacing is performed by replacing the hip joint with a metal cup in the acetabulum that articulates with a bearing that is capped on the prepared femoral head. Typically, the cap has a small stem that goes down the neck of the femur, and the procedure does not involve the placement of a stem down the shaft of the femoral diaphysis. This feature allows for easier component placement in those who have deformities associated with Perthes disease of the proximal femur from prior surgeries, such as coxa vara or coxa valga.[2,3] These metal-on-metal designs are usually larger in diameter than most THA components, which have the potential to decrease the risk of dislocation rates that may occur more frequently in these younger, more-active patients.[4,5] In addition, this procedure is more bone conserving than a THA because it preserves the proximal femur, which may allow for an easier revision to a THA, if necessary.[6–8]

Several reports on resurfacings have shown excellent results in patients younger than 40 years with reported survivorships of 93% or greater.[4,9–13]

No funding was received in support for the publication of this article. The authors have nothing to disclose in direct relation to the work submitted in this article.
Center for Joint Preservation and Replacement, Rubin Institute for Advanced Orthopedics, Sinai Hospital of Baltimore, 401 West Belvedere Avenue, Baltimore, MD 21215, USA
* Corresponding author.
E-mail addresses: mmont@lifebridgehealth.org; rhondamont@aol.com

Orthop Clin N Am 42 (2011) 419–422
doi:10.1016/j.ocl.2011.04.002
0030-5898/11/$ – see front matter © 2011 Elsevier Inc. All rights reserved.

Boyd and colleagues[14] reported on 18 patients (19 hips) who underwent total hip resurfacing for Legg-Calvé-Perthes disease; they observed a 100% survivorship at a mean follow-up of 51 months (range, 26–72 months) and noted that 18 of the 19 hips had good to excellent clinical results as evidenced by Harris hip scores of 80 points or more. The investigators concluded that their results for resurfacing compared similarly to other studies using standard THA. Amstutz and colleagues[9] studied 21 patients (25 hips) who had a mean age of 38 years (range, 18–57 years) and underwent resurfacing for Legg-Calvé-Perthes disease (14 hips) or slipped capital femoral epiphysis (11 hips). At a mean follow-up of 4.7 years (range, 2.7–8.1 years), they observed a 92% survivorship.

There are a few contraindications to total hip resurfacing. Although wear rates seen with metal-on-metal bearings are extremely low, there have been reports of increased metal ion concentrations in these patients.[15,16] Therefore, renal dysfunction is an absolute contraindication to this procedure because metal ions are excreted by the kidneys.[6] In addition, because the effect of increased metal ions is mostly unknown, the US Food and Drug Administration recommends that women of child-bearing age should not undergo this procedure. Other relative contraindications to this procedure are the presence of extensive cystic damage of the femoral head or severe osteoporosis because a healthy bone stock is important for good component fixation and sizing. Intraoperative assessment should be made of the femoral head, and the authors recommend that if less than 75% of the

bone is viable, a standard THA should be performed. A report from the Australian Orthopaedic Association National Joint Replacement registry noted a higher failure rate in total hip resurfacing than in THA in patients with acetabular cup sizes less than 50 mm,[17] which may have implications for smaller patients who have had Perthes disease. Complications that have been reported with this procedure include local adverse tissue reactions such as pseudotumor and aseptic lymphocytic vasculitis–associated lesions, although symptomatic lesions seem to occur in less than 1% of all patients undergoing the procedure. The true incidence and cause of these complications is unknown.[18,19]

Total hip resurfacing is a technically demanding procedure, and it is recommended that it be performed only by an experienced surgeon.[20] Patients who had Legg-Calvé-Perthes disease may have unique deformities that necessitate variations in the surgical approach. These patients often have overgrowth of bone around the femoral head (coxa magna) or flattening of the femoral head (coxa plana) and thus are at an increased risk for limb length shortening and femoral neck impingement after the procedure.[6,21,22] One must focus on not notching the femoral neck when preparing these hips with deformed femoral heads. Trochanteric advancement is a useful variation to this procedure, described by Boyd and colleagues,[14] to prevent these complications. The greater trochanter is cut and advanced over the femoral neck under the vastus lateralis muscle. The bone is then fixed with 2 cables, one placed over the greater trochanter and the other through 2 drill

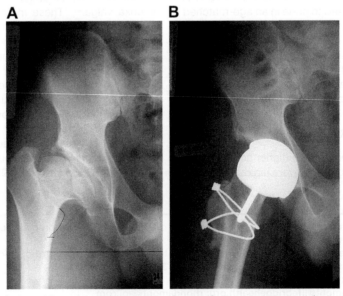

Fig. 1. Total hip resurfacing with trochanteric osteotomy for significant coxa magna and coxa plana (A) in a 30-year-old woman who had hip pain for more than 10 years after Legg-Calvé-Perthes disease (B).

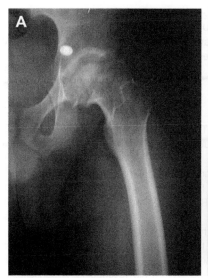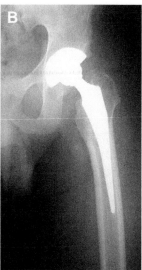

Fig. 2. Radiographs before (*A*) and after (*B*) a THA in a 16-year-old adolescent boy with hip pain for 3 years after resolved Legg-Calvé-Perthes disease.

holes in the cortex of the femoral neck to aid in compression (**Fig. 1**). This mode of fixing adds length to the femoral neck to counter limb length discrepancies and tightens the abductor muscle group for later increased strength.

THA

In patients who are poor candidates for a resurfacing, a standard THA may be performed (**Fig. 2**). There are only a few published reports on exclusive cohorts of patients undergoing THA for residual arthritis from Legg-Calvé-Perthes disease. However, survivorship of this procedure in young adults has ranged from 51% to 94% at midterm follow-up in reports, including patients who have diagnoses of Legg-Calvé-Perthes disease.[23–28] Since the publication of these articles, advancements in polyethylene bearings and femoral stems have further increased THA implant survivorship and durability, making these procedures even more palatable to younger patients. One recent study of the Danish Hip Registry found in 361 patients (404 hips) who had Legg-Calvé-Perthes disease and had undergone THA, a revision rate of only 6% (24 of 404 hips) at a mean follow-up of 4.6 years (range, 1 day–12 years).[24] It was noted that patients undergoing THA who previously had Legg-Calvé-Perthes disease were at no increased risk for revision when matched to other patient cohorts. Another study from the Norwegian Arthroplasty Registry of patients who underwent THA for either Legg-Calvé-Perthes disease or epiphysiolysis derived a Kaplan-Meier 10-year survivorship of 92% (55 revisions in 708 hips).[23] The mean age at the time of surgery was 52 years (range, 15–88 years).

Total hip arthroplasties differ from resurfacing in that they are more commonly performed with a smaller metal head that articulates in an acetabular cup between a polyethylene liner. Variations exist such as using ceramic material on both the head and neck as the articulating surface, which has been shown to have extremely low wear rates.[29,30] One of the main differences between THA and resurfacing is that in the former, the entire femoral head and neck are removed and a stem is placed down the proximal diaphysis of the femur. This can make the procedure technically demanding in patients with coxa vara or coxa valga deformities from previous femoral osteotomy procedures as children, and occasionally, an osteotomy needs to be combined with the THA to restore the anatomy. Patients may also have extensive scar tissue from prior procedures, which may make exposure and hip preparation difficult.

Postsurgical rehabilitation is similar for THA and resurfacing. Patients are initially seen in the hospital for daily physical therapy. Typically, patients are kept at 50% partial weight bearing for the first 6 weeks after surgery while undergoing outpatient rehabilitation, during which they work on strengthening exercises. They are then allowed to advance to weight bearing as tolerated.

SUMMARY

The treatment of patients who have arthritis after the treatment of Legg-Calvé-Perthes disease requires special consideration for the joint arthroplasty surgeon. These patients are younger, active, and may have a marked deformity of the femoral head, neck, or proximal shaft. Total hip resurfacing offers some potential advantages in that it is bone preserving. Standard THA has excellent results with newer component designs and materials and offers a promising treatment option for these patients as well.

REFERENCES

1. Froberg L, Christensen F, Pedersen NW, et al. The need for THA in Perthes disease: a long-term study. Clin Orthop Relat Res 2011;469(4):1134–40.

2. Clohisy JC, Keeney JA, Schoenecker PL. Preliminary assessment and treatment guidelines for hip disorders in young adults. Clin Orthop Relat Res 2005;441:168.

3. Herring JA, Kim HT, Browne H. Legg-Calve-Perthes disease. Part II: prospective multicenter study of the effect of treatment on outcome. J Bone Joint Surg Am 2004;86:2121.

4. Mont MA, Seyler TM, Marker DR, et al. Use of metal-on-metal total hip resurfacing for the treatment of osteonecrosis of the femoral head. J Bone Joint Surg Am 2006;88(Suppl 3):90.

5. Lieske S, John M, Rimasch C, et al. [Dislocation as a rare complication of resurfacing of the hip joint. Case report and meta-analysis]. Unfallchirurg 2008;111:637 [in German].

6. Amstutz HC, Beaule PE, Dorey FJ, et al. Metal-on-metal hybrid surface arthroplasty. Surgical Technique. J Bone Joint Surg Am 2006;88(Suppl 1 Pt 2):234.

7. Ballard WT, Lowry DA, Brand RA. Resection arthroplasty of the hip. J Arthroplasty 1995;10:772.

8. Mont MA, McGrath MS, Ulrich SD, et al. Metal-on-metal total hip resurfacing arthroplasty in the presence of extra-articular deformities or implants. J Bone Joint Surg Am 2008;90(Suppl 3):45.

9. Amstutz HC, Su EP, Le Duff MJ. Surface arthroplasty in young patients with hip arthritis secondary to childhood disorders. Orthop Clin North Am 2005;36:223.

10. Amstutz HC, Le Duff MJ. Hip resurfacing results for osteonecrosis are as good as for other etiologies at 2 to 12 years. Clin Orthop Relat Res 2010; 468:375.

11. Beaule PE, Amstutz HC, Le Duff M, et al. Surface arthroplasty for osteonecrosis of the hip: hemiresurfacing versus metal-on-metal hybrid resurfacing. J Arthroplasty 2004;19:54.

12. Aulakh TS, Rao C, Kuiper JH, et al. Hip resurfacing and osteonecrosis: results from an independent hip resurfacing register. Arch Orthop Trauma Surg 2010;130:841.

13. Revell MP, McBryde CW, Bhatnagar S, et al. Metal-on-metal hip resurfacing in osteonecrosis of the femoral head. J Bone Joint Surg Am 2006;88(Suppl 3):98.

14. Boyd HS, Ulrich SD, Seyler TM, et al. Resurfacing for Perthes disease: an alternative to standard hip arthroplasty. Clin Orthop Relat Res 2007;465:80.

15. Back DL, Young DA, Shimmin AJ. How do serum cobalt and chromium levels change after metal-on-metal hip resurfacing? Clin Orthop Relat Res 2005; 438:177.

16. Vendittoli PA, Mottard S, Roy AG, et al. Chromium and cobalt ion release following the Durom high carbon content, forged metal-on-metal surface replacement of the hip. J Bone Joint Surg Br 2007;89:441.

17. Prosser GH, Yates PJ, Wood DJ, et al. Outcome of primary resurfacing hip replacement: evaluation of risk factors for early revision. Acta Orthop 2010;81:66.

18. Glyn-Jones S, Pandit H, Kwon YM, et al. Risk factors for inflammatory pseudotumour formation following hip resurfacing. J Bone Joint Surg Br 2009;91:1566.

19. O'Neill M, Beaule PE, Bin Nasser A, et al. Canadian academic experience with metal-on-metal hip resurfacing. Bull NYU Hosp Jt Dis 2009;67:128.

20. De Smet K, Campbell PA, Gill HS. Metal-on-metal hip resurfacing: a consensus from the Advanced Hip Resurfacing Course, Ghent, 2009. J Bone Joint Surg Br 2010;92:335.

21. Eilert RE, Hill K, Bach J. Greater trochanteric transfer for the treatment of coxa brevis. Clin Orthop Relat Res 2005;434:92.

22. Schneidmueller D, Carstens C, Thomsen M. Surgical treatment of overgrowth of the greater trochanter in children and adolescents. J Pediatr Orthop 2006;26:486.

23. Furnes O, Lie SA, Espehaug B, et al. Hip disease and the prognosis of total hip replacements. A review of 53,698 primary total hip replacements reported to the Norwegian Arthroplasty Register 1987–99. J Bone Joint Surg Br 2001;83:579.

24. Thillemann TM, Pedersen AB, Johnsen SP, et al. Implant survival after primary THA due to childhood hip disorders: results from the Danish Hip Arthroplasty Registry. Acta Orthop 2008;79:769.

25. Wangen H, Lereim P, Holm I, et al. Hip arthroplasty in patients younger than 30 years: excellent ten to 16-year follow-up results with a HA-coated stem. Int Orthop 2008;32:203.

26. Clohisy JC, Oryhon JM, Seyler TM, et al. Function and fixation of THA in patients 25 years of age or younger. Clin Orthop Relat Res 2010;468:3207.

27. Sayeed SA, Johnson AJ, Stroh DA, et al. Hip resurfacing in patients who have osteonecrosis and are 25 years or under. Clin Orthop Relat Res 2010. [Epub ahead of print].

28. Restrepo C, Lettich T, Roberts N, et al. Uncemented THA in patients less than twenty-years. Acta Orthop Belg 2008;74:615.

29. Jazrawi LM, Bogner E, Della Valle CJ, et al. Wear rates of ceramic-on-ceramic bearing surfaces in total hip implants: a 12-year follow-up study. J Arthroplasty 1999;14:781.

30. Capello WN, D'Antonio JA, Feinberg JR, et al. Ceramic-on-ceramic THA: update. J Arthroplasty 2008;23:39.

Future Biologic Treatments for Perthes Disease

David G. Little, MBBS, FRACS(Orth), PhD[a,b,]*,
Harry K.W. Kim, MD, MSc, FRCSC[c,d]

KEYWORDS

- Perthes disease • Experimental strategies
- Biologic interventions

Current nonoperative treatment for Perthes disease, Scottish Rite orthosis, does not seem to affect outcome.[1,2] The effects of surgical treatments, such as a femoral varus osteotomy and the Salter's innominate osteotomy, also had moderate effects in the multicenter prospective study by Herring and colleagues. For example, in lateral pillar B hips greater than age 8 years where the effect of surgery was greatest, the rate of spherical hips increased from 44% to 73%.[3] This means that in this favorable scenario, while 29% of the patients operated gained a spherical hip that would not have occurred in the natural evolution of the disease, 71% of patients did not benefit, as 44% would have had a spherical head anyway, and 27% did not achieve sphericity even with surgery. While the effects of surgery are definite, they are by no means universally positive.

PATHOLOGY OF PERTHES DISEASE

Perthes disease can be defined as idiopathic avascular necrosis of the femoral head in childhood. The initiating insult triggering the onset of Perthes disease remains unknown, making a true description of the pathology difficult. However, a great deal more is known about Perthes disease pathogenesis, much of which has been gained by correlating the few true histologic specimens with radiographs, and also by examining animal models of Perthes disease. Although trauma may play a part in Perthes disease, it is unlikely to be the only factor, as traumatic avascular necrosis often behaves differently from Perthes disease. In truth, the initiating factor remains unknown.

However, what is clear is that the femoral head blood supply is very dependent on the ascending branches of the lateral femoral circumflex, in turn a branch of profunda femoris. A condition very similar but not identical to Perthes can be created in piglets by tying off these and other ascending vessels, along with the repetitive loading of the hip joint.[4] In Perthes disease, it is well known that the bone age is delayed, an average of 2 years in girls and 1 year in boys.[3] This means the amount of cartilage present in the developing femoral head is larger and the ossific nucleus smaller. In one theory, these vessels have to traverse a larger-than-normal cartilaginous anlage to get to the epiphysis and are thus vulnerable to mechanical

Funding sources: Dr Little: NHMRC, Orthopaedic Research Fund, Novartis Pharma; Dr Kim: Shriners Hospitals for Children, POSNA, OREF, Roche.

Conflict of Interest: Dr Little: Previously Consultant for Novartis Pharma, Dr Kim: nil.

[a] Department of Orthopaedics, Orthopaedic Research, The Children's Hospital at Westmead, Locked Bag 4001, Westmead, NSW 2145, Australia

[b] Discipline of Paediatrics and Child Health, University of Sydney, Sydney, NSW 2006, Australia

[c] Center for Excellence in Hip Disorders, Research Department, Texas Scottish Rite Hospital for Children, 2222 Welborn Street, Dallas, TX 75219, USA

[d] Department of Orthopedic Surgery, University of Texas Southwestern Medical Center, 1801 Inwood Road, WA4.312, Dallas, TX 75390, USA

* Corresponding author. Department of Orthopaedics, The Children's Hospital at Westmead, Locked Bag 4001, Westmead, NSW 2145, Australia.

E-mail address: DavidL3@chw.edu.au

orthopedic.theclinics.com

compression.[5] A particular strain of rat called the SHR rat also has a delayed bone age and the onset of a Perthes-like condition occurs in 50% of male rats that stand on their hind limbs to feed.[6] When these rats are prevented from weight bearing, avascular necrosis does not occur.

The few human specimens available show an enlarged cartilaginous anlage, fibrocartilaginous and fibrovascular proliferation, and a disorganization of the growth plate.[7,8] Depending where the biopsy is taken, areas of granulation tissue or endochondral ossification can be seen. Some of the new bone that has managed to form can be seen to be reinfarcted.

The stages of Perthes disease are well accepted: (1) initial, (2) fragmentation, (3) reossification, and (4) healed. In the initial phase, the ossific nucleus is not growing due to the avascular necrosis, but the cartilaginous anlage continues to enlarge, receiving nutrition from the synovial fluid. Next the femoral head starts to collapse. The pathology here (at least from animal models) is that osteoclasts are removing the dead bone.[4] Resorptive phase may be a better term for this stage than fragmentation. There is an uncoupling of the normal bone remodeling mechanism whereby bone resorption is followed by bone formation. This gives the appearance on radiographs of a central sequestrum that continues to mineralize and is dense,[9] and surrounding lytic areas yet to ossify. Eventually the neo-cartilage in the femoral head undergoes endochondral ossification with the invasion of blood vessels followed by osteoblasts. Eventually all the dead bone is removed and replaced with new bone. This bone is then remodeled into lamellar bone, and the process is complete. However, it is important to note that the lag between resorption and formation leave the largely cartilaginous head very soft and subject to the deformation of the loads placed on it.

Finally, the circulation re-establishes itself, and ossification proceeds from lateral to medial and posterior to anterior. Shape changes continue to occur during the remodeling phase; these can be either beneficial or harmful.[10]

Magnetic resonance imaging (MRI) studies of Perthes disease attest to significant inflammatory changes in the synovium and ligamentum teres, contributing to subluxation.[11,12]

HYPOTHESES GENERATED FROM RADIOLOGICAL AND PATHOPHYSIOLOGICAL FINDINGS
Inflammatory Changes

The inflammatory changes in Perthes disease are most marked during the fragmentation phase (**Fig. 1**). As this phase is when bone resorption and bone formation are uncoupled, it may be that inflammatory mediators are inhibiting bone formation. Such phenomena are well known to disturb the anabolic/catabolic balance in rheumatoid arthritis.[13] Osteoblasts cannot differentiate from mesenchymal stem cells in the presence of high levels cytokines such as tumor necrosis factor (TNF)-α and interleukin (I1-β).[14] If the phathophysiological mechanisms are similar, controlling inflammation may play some role in encouraging new bone formation as well as decreasing bone resorption.

Bone Resorption

While eventual resorption of the necrotic sequestrum would be necessary to restore the normal mechanical properties of the femoral head, rapid resorption leads to collapse. A great deal of research has been performed looking at the role of bisphosphonates in models of Perthes disease. In rodent traumatic models, femoral head structure can be almost completely preserved with zoledronic acid or alendronate treatment.[15,16] In the SHR model, zoledronic acid can improve femoral head shape.[17]

In the piglet model of ischemic necrosis where the femoral head vessels are disrupted by a ligature,

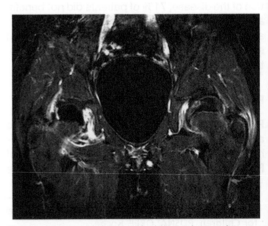

Fig. 1. 9-year-old boy with bilateral asynchronous Legg-Calvé-Perthes (LCP) disease.[12] 2-dimensional T1-weighted spoiled gradient-recalled echo fat-saturated contrast-enhanced subtraction image shows nonenhancement of entire right femoral head and extensive right hip joint synovitis. Note heterogeneous enhancement of left proximal femoral epiphysis and left hip synovitis as well. Magnetic resonance imaging findings support diagnosis of bilateral LCP disease, with right hip in necrotic phase and left hip likely in revascularization phase. (*From* Dillman JR, Hernandez RJ. MRI of Legg-Calve-Perthes disease. AJR Am J Roentgenol 2009;193:1402; with permission.)

systemic ibandronate significantly improves the maintenance of femoral head shape.[18] However, the biodistribution of bisphosphonate to the necrotic bone is initially poor, favoring local delivery.[19,20] Treatment with an inhibitor of RANKL, osteoprotegerin (OPG), was systemically effective but also had major effects on growth plate remodelling.[21]

In small animal models, the return of bone formation is rapid with bisphosphonate therapy. However, this finding is not observed in the piglet model or in patients with Perthes disease. This

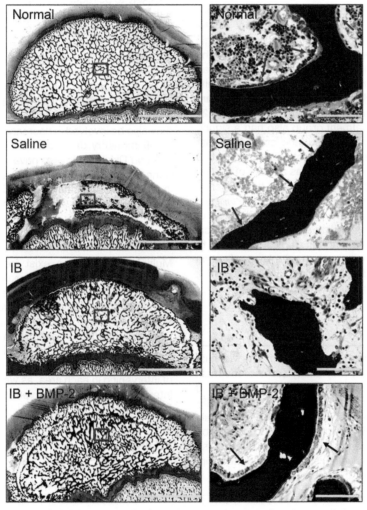

Fig. 2. Histologic sections of the femoral heads from the normal, saline, ibandronate (IB), and the combined IB plus BMP-2 groups.[24] The representative histologic sections were stained with von Kossa and McNeal tetrachrome. The left panels show low magnification views of the epiphyses (bars: 1.0 cm), and boxed areas in the left panels are magnified and shown in the right panels (bars: 100 μm). The femoral head from the saline group shows trabecular bone resorption and a collapsed femoral head structure, while the femoral heads from the IB and the IB + BMP-2 groups show preservation of the trabecular bone and the spherical femoral head structure. Note the head-within-head appearance seen in the IB plus BMP-2 group with thickened trabeculae in the central region of the head. The right panels show osteoblasts lining the trabecular bone surface in the normal group (*red arrows*), while osteoblasts are absent in the saline group (*blue arrows*). In the IB group, osteoblasts are also absent. In contrast, osteoblasts lining the trabecular bone are seen in the IB plus BMP-2 group (*black arrows*), similar to the normal group. (*From* Vandermeer J, Kamiya N, Aya-ay J, et al. Local administration of ibandronate and bone morphogenetic protein-2 stimulates bone formation and decreases femoral head deformity following ischemic osteonecrosis of the immature femoral head. J Bone Joint Surg Am 2011;93:905–13; with permission.)

suggests that while anticatabolic strategies are likely to be necessary to preserve femoral head shape, stimulation of bone formation is likely to be also desirable.

Bone Formation

An anabolic strategy would increase revascularization and couple this with increased bone formation. Bone morphogenic proteins (BMPs) and bisphosphonates are known to be synergistic in bone repair.[22,23] In the piglet model, this experimental strategy used BMP-2 injection at the same time as local ibandronate infusion as a single intraosseous injection.[24] Compared with the control group, the combined therapy group had a significant decrease in femoral head deformity and the osteoclast number and a significant increase in the trabecular bone volume (**Fig. 2**). The combined treatment group also had a significantly higher osteoblast surface compared with the local ibandronate treatment group, suggesting an increased bone formation as a result of adding BMP-2. One cautionary finding was the presence of heterotopic ossification in the hip joint capsule. This was postulated to be due to a leakage of BMP-2 into the joint during and following the local injection procedure. Further studies underway to determine whether the heterotopic ossification can be prevented by lowering the dose of BMP-2 and changing the delivery technique.

FUTURE DIRECTIONS
Inflammation

Further MRI studies and sampling of synovial fluid during arthrography may clarify some of the main inflammatory mediators in Perthes disease. If particular inflammatory markers such as TNF-α are identified, current treatments used in juvenile rheumatoid arthritis such as infliximab could be considered. Decreasing inflammation may also have a role in reducing subluxation of the hip, another factor in the genesis of deformity in Perthes disease.

Bone Resorption

Local delivery of bisphosphonates into the femoral head has been investigated but requires further study. Denosumab, an antibody to RANKL, profoundly inhibits bone resorption by interrupting osteoclastogenesis. This approach would obviate the need for the drug to circulate into the necrotic bone, but the systemic effects of the drug are likely to be marked. Other anticatabolic agents that have shorter half-lives could also be considered, especially via local sustained delivery. Such drugs

include cathepsin K inhibitors, as well as novel experimental agents such as inhibitor of NF-B kinases (IKK) inhibitors and inhibitors of the osteoclast vacuolar adenosine triphosphatase (ATPase) and chloride channels of the osteoclast.[25–27]

Bone Formation

While local delivery of BMPs may be feasible, they are expensive agents, and special delivery systems are likely to be required to avoid heterotopic ossification in the joint. Other novel anabolic agents are emerging, particularly those working via the Wnt pathway, a powerful modulator of bone remodeling. Sclerostin antibody in people simultaneously increases bone formation while reducing markers of bone resorption.[28] TNF-α induces expression of another osteoblast inhibitor, Dkk1, which also regulates sclerostin,[29,30] and these mediators may also be involved in decreasing bone formation in inflammatory disorders.[31] Antibodies to sclerostin and Dkk1 would also have systemic effect on bone formation, but their half-lives are likely to be in the order of months, such that these effects should reverse after a period of washout.

SUMMARY

Multiple opportunities exist for pharmaceutical/biologic intervention in the areas of inflammation, bone resorption, and bone formation, all of which are among the factors that create subluxation and femoral head deformity in Perthes disease. Reaching the goal of effective medical treatment for Perthes disease will require a systematic research endeavor to define and explore the effect of intervening in each area, as well as exploring the interaction of these interventions with surgical treatment.

REFERENCES

1. Martinez AG, Weinstein SL, Dietz FR. The weight-bearing abduction brace for the treatment of Legg-Perthes disease. J Bone Joint Surg Am 1992;74(1):12–21.
2. Wiig O, Terjesen T, Svenningsen S. Prognostic factors and outcome of treatment in Perthes' disease: a prospective study of 368 patients with five-year follow-up. J Bone Joint Surg Br 2008;90(10):1364–71.
3. Herring JA, Kim HT, Browne R. Legg-Calve-Perthes disease. Part II: prospective multicenter study of the effect of treatment on outcome. J Bone Joint Surg Am 2004;86(10):2121–34.
4. Kim HK, Su PH. Development of flattening and apparent fragmentation following ischemic necrosis

of the capital femoral epiphysis in a piglet model. J Bone Joint Surg Am 2002;84(8):1329–34.

5. Ponseti IV. Legg-Perthes disease; observations on pathological changes in two cases. J Bone Joint Surg Am 1956;38(4):739–50.

6. Suehiro M, Hirano I, Mihara K, et al. Etiologic factors in femoral head osteonecrosis in growing rats. J Orthop Sci 2000;5(1):52–6.

7. Catterall A, Pringle J, Byers PD, et al. A review of the morphology of Perthes' disease. J Bone Joint Surg Br 1982;64(3):269–75.

8. Ponseti IV, Maynard JA, Weinstein SL, et al. Legg-Calve-Perthes disease. Histochemical and ultrastructural observations of the epiphyseal cartilage and physis. J Bone Joint Surg Am 1983;65(6): 797–807.

9. Hofstaetter JG, Roschger P, Klaushofer K, et al. Increased matrix mineralization in the immature femoral head following ischemic osteonecrosis. Bone 2010;46(2):379–85.

10. Herring JA, Williams JJ, Neustadt JN, et al. Evolution of femoral head deformity during the healing phase of Legg-Calve-Perthes disease. J Pediatr Orthop 1993;13(1):41–5.

11. Hochbergs P, Eckerwall G, Egund N, et al. Synovitis in Legg-Calve-Perthes disease. Evaluation with MR imaging in 84 hips. Acta Radiol 1998;39(5):532–7.

12. Dillman JR, Hernandez RJ. MRI of Legg-Calve-Perthes disease. AJR Am J Roentgenol 2009; 193(5):1394–407.

13. Choi Y, Arron JR, Townsend MJ. Promising bone-related therapeutic targets for rheumatoid arthritis. Nat Rev Rheumatol 2009;5(10):543–8.

14. Lacey DC, Simmons PJ, Graves SE, et al. Proinflammatory cytokines inhibit osteogenic differentiation from stem cells: implications for bone repair during inflammation. Osteoarthritis Cartilage 2009;17(6):735–42.

15. Little DG, Peat RA, McEvoy A, et al. Zoledronic acid treatment results in retention of femoral head structure after traumatic osteonecrosis in young Wistar rats. J Bone Miner Res 2003;18(11):2016–22.

16. Peled E, Bejar J, Zinman C, et al. Alendronate preserves femoral head shape and height/length ratios in an experimental rat model: a computer-assisted analysis. Indian J Orthop 2009;43(1):22–6.

17. Little DG, McDonald M, Sharpe IT, et al. Zoledronic acid improves femoral head sphericity in a rat model of perthes disease. J Orthop Res 2005; 23(4):862–8.

18. Kim HK, Randall TS, Bian H, et al. Ibandronate for prevention of femoral head deformity after ischemic necrosis of the capital femoral epiphysis in immature pigs. J Bone Joint Surg Am 2005;87(3):550–7.

19. Kim HK, Sanders M, Athavale S, et al. Local bioavailability and distribution of systemically (parenterally)

administered ibandronate in the infarcted femoral head. Bone 2006;39(1):205–12.

20. Aya-ay J, Athavale S, Morgan-Bagley S, et al. Retention, distribution, and effects of intraosseously administered ibandronate in the infarcted femoral head. J Bone Miner Res 2007;22(1):93–100.

21. Kim HK, Morgan-Bagley S, Kostenuik P. RANKL inhibition: a novel strategy to decrease femoral head deformity after ischemic osteonecrosis. J Bone Miner Res 2006;21(12):1946–54.

22. Little DG, McDonald M, Bransford R, et al. Manipulation of the anabolic and catabolic responses with OP-1 and zoledronic acid in a rat critical defect model. J Bone Miner Res 2005;20(11):2044–52.

23. Harding AK, Aspenberg P, Kataoka M, et al. Manipulating the anabolic and catabolic response in bone graft remodeling: synergism by a combination of local BMP-7 and a single systemic dose of zoledronate. J Orthop Res 2008;26(9):1245–9.

24. Vandermeer J, Kamiya N, Aya-ay J, et al. Local administration of ibandronate and bone morphogenetic protein-2 stimulates bone formation and decreases femoral head deformity following ischemic osteonecrosis of the immature femoral head. J Bone Joint Surg Am, in press.

25. Reid IR. Anti-resorptive therapies for osteoporosis. Semin Cell Dev Biol 2008;19(5):473–8.

26. Schaller S, Henriksen K, Sveigaard C, et al. The chloride channel inhibitor NS3736 [corrected] prevents bone resorption in ovariectomized rats without changing bone formation. J Bone Miner Res 2004;19(7):1144–53.

27. Sorensen MG, Henriksen K, Neutzsky-Wulff AV, et al. Diphyllin, a novel and naturally potent V-ATPase inhibitor, abrogates acidification of the osteoclastic resorption lacunae and bone resorption. J Bone Miner Res 2007;22(10):1640–8.

28. Padhi D, Jang G, Stouch B, et al. Single-dose, placebo-controlled, randomized study of AMG 785, a sclerostin monoclonal antibody. J Bone Miner Res 2011;26(1):19–26.

29. Heiland GR, Zwerina K, Baum W, et al. Neutralisation of Dkk-1 protects from systemic bone loss during inflammation and reduces sclerostin expression. Ann Rheum Dis 2010;69(12):2152–9.

30. Vincent C, Findlay DM, Welldon KJ, et al. Proinflammatory cytokines TNF-related weak inducer of apoptosis (TWEAK) and TNFalpha induce the mitogen-activated protein kinase (MAPK)-dependent expression of sclerostin in human osteoblasts. J Bone Miner Res 2009;24(8):1434–49.

31. Walsh NC, Reinwald S, Manning CA, et al. Osteoblast function is compromised at sites of focal bone erosion in inflammatory arthritis. J Bone Miner Res 2009;24(9):1572–85.

Core Decompression for Juvenile Osteonecrosis

José A. Herrera-Soto, MD[a],*, Charles T. Price, MD[a,b]

KEYWORDS

- Core decompression • Avascular necrosis
- Legg-Calvé-Perthes disease • Femoral head
- Osteonecrosis

When Legg-Calvé-Perthes disease (LCPD) develops at age 12 years or older, the results are generally poor, with or without current methods of treatment.[1–5] These juvenile patients are more likely to become Stulberg class V even when the necrotic segment is less than 50% of the femoral head.[1,4] Joseph and colleagues[1] reported 62 patients aged 12 years or older at onset. In their series, neither the Catterall group nor the Herring grade correlated with final outcome and none benefited from containment treatment.

We propose the term idiopathic juvenile osteonecrosis to distinguish this age group from younger children with Perthes disease and from adults with osteonecrosis of the femoral head. One difference is that the femoral head in the older pediatric age group does not reconstitute as rapidly as in younger children with LCPD.[6] Another difference between juvenile osteonecrosis and younger children with Perthes disease it that the older age group has less remodeling capacity of the femoral head or acetabulum.[1,2,5,7]

Compared with adults, juvenile osteonecrosis may have a slightly more favorable prognosis. In adults, the rate of bone resorption exceeds the rate of bone deposition.[8] This difference causes a weakness in the structural integrity of the bone followed by subchondral fracture and collapse.[9]

Ficat[10] identified that stage III osteonecrosis in adults is associated with a break in the articular surface. However, there is a transitional stage in which a subchondral fracture may be present without segmental collapse.[10] Young children have thick articular cartilage that may be more resistant to deformation and disruption than that of older children. Adolescents may also tolerate some subsidence of the necrotic fragment without disruption of the articular surface. Restoring support to the joint surface before cartilage fracture may preserve joint function.[11]

The treatment rationale of the femoral head should be tailored to address these differences between adult and childhood osteonecrosis of the femoral head. Joseph and colleagues[1] suggested that an alternative method of treatment of juvenile osteonecrosis should be investigated. He concluded that the success of treatment depends on necrotic bone resorption (elimination), new bone formation in its place, and a remodeling process that is protected from further deformation by adequate containment. It is our opinion that early core decompression combined with containment in the form of a shelf acetabuloplasty can meet these objectives and may improve outcomes compared with the natural history and with previous treatment methods for this age group. Core

The authors have no financial conflicts of interest.

[a] Division of Pediatric Orthopedics, The Arnold Palmer Hospital for Children, 83 West Columbia Street, Orlando, FL 32806, USA

[b] Orthopedic Surgery, University of Central Florida College of Medicine, 6850 Lake Nona Boulevard, Orlando, FL 32827, USA

* Corresponding author.

E-mail address: jose.herrera@orlandohealth.com

Orthop Clin N Am 42 (2011) 429–436

doi:10.1016/j.ocl.2011.04.004

decompression and shelf acetabuloplasty (labral support) for idiopathic juvenile osteonecrosis is the focus of this article.

CORE DECOMPRESSION

Core decompression was reported as a possible solution for LCPD in the 1930s.[12,13] Details and examples of cases were not described, but Ferguson and Howorth[13] indicated that drilling in the active stage resulted in earlier and more complete healing.

The objectives of core decompression are to remove necrotic bone, reduce venous congestion, and encourage revascularization.[14] Removal of necrotic bone has been identified as a key component for success of core decompression.[15,16] Some investigators advocate arthroscopic inspection to ensure removal of necrotic bone.[17,18]

The principle objective of decompression is to reduce intraosseous pressure to decrease venous congestion and improve capillary blood flow. The bone marrow pressure in the femoral head and neck is increased in patients who develop osteonecrosis.[10,19] The pressure is reduced and venous flow improved in some patients following decompression by drilling or by proximal femoral osteotomy.[19,20] Vascularity of the proximal femur is also enhanced by the angiogenesis caused by the trephine opening new vascular channels. In children, the growth plate of the proximal femur is a barrier to revascularization.[21] Reossification of the femoral head is facilitated by removal or fenestration of the epiphyseal plate.[21] Thus, core decompression has several beneficial effects for revascularization of the femoral head.

Numerous investigators have compared core decompression with nonoperative management for osteonecrosis of the femoral head. Improved outcomes have been noted following core decompression in the early stages of necrosis.[15,16,22–27] Fairbank and colleagues[25] reported satisfactory long-term results of core decompression performed in Ficat stages I and II (**Fig. 1**). Ficat and Arlet[28] classified patients with a crescent sign as stage II. Stage III indicates flattening and collapse of the femoral head. Other investigators have included the crescent sign as stage III with or without femoral head collapse.[29]

Techniques for core decompression have ranged from multiple small drillings with 3.2-mm Steinmann pins[30,31] to expanding reamers and trapdoor procedures that remove large amounts of necrotic bone.[14] Small pin drillings have been less effective for larger lesions with higher intraosseous pressures.[19] More complete removal of necrotic bone has been recommended for larger lesions in later stages of disease, including stage III, as long as the articular cartilage is intact.[14]

Maintaining a sturdy structural support in the decompressed area during the revascularization process helps prevent disruption of the articular cartilage.[15,16,32] Gradual substitution of necrotic bone or implant material by living bone keeps the decline of the bone's mechanical properties to a minimum.[33] Various graft materials and adjunctive techniques have been used following core decompression.[16,34,35] Liebermann and colleagues[36] and Chang and colleagues[37] performed core decompressions with bone grafting and partially purified bone morphogenic proteins as adjuncts. Keizer and colleagues[16] noted improved outcomes with autograft compared with allograft. For patients with Ficat stage III necrosis, free vascularized fibular grafting is beneficial.[35] Free vascularized fibular grafting in children and adolescents for stage III osteonecrosis has better reported outcomes than those performed in adults.[38]

In the adult population, the prognosis depends on several factors, including the size of the lesion, the location, and the bone quality of the uninvolved portion of the femoral head.[31,39–45] The smaller the lesion, the better the result, regardless of whether it is Ficat stage I or II.[31,39–41] Koo and Kim[43] reported that patients with less than 30% of femoral head involvement did not develop progression of the osteonecrosis, whereas all the hips with more than 40% involvement collapsed. The location of involvement of hip osteonecrosis is also an important factor.[41] Lateral lesions fare worse compared with those with medial or lateral involvement.[31] These factors also apply to juvenile osteonecrosis but the adolescent age group with open growth plates may have a more favorable prognosis when treated later in the course of disease.

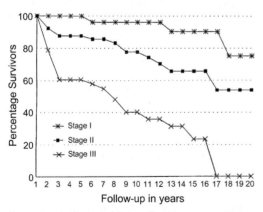

Fig. 1. Survival curves for each Ficat stage. (*Reproduced from* Fairbank AC, Bhatia D, Jennah RH, et al. Long-term results of core decompression for ischaemic necrosis of the femoral head. J Bone Joint Surg Br 1995;77:47; with permission.)

Several investigators identified that the femoral epiphyseal height is unlikely to improve after collapse.[7,15] Femoral head flattening has also been found to be a prognostic factor in the adult population.[15,45,46] These investigators recommended that surgery should be performed as early as possible to prevent collapse.[47,48] However, even in the presence of femoral head collapse, core decompression may help relieve pain.[15,49]

SURGICAL TECHNIQUE

The critical component for performing an adequate core decompression is to place the trephine in the center of the necrotic defect as close as possible to the articular surface (Fig. 2A, B), although this does not mean the center of the femoral head. We prefer to perform the procedure on a radiolucent table and drape the lower extremity free to be able to manipulate the limb and verify the guidewire position. Recently, a lateral decubitus position has been the preferred method.

The guidewire and trephine are inserted proximal to the level of the lesser trochanter to minimize the risk of subtrochanteric fracture from the stress riser created by the core tunnel. Once the guide is properly placed, the trephine is advanced. Trephines that are from 8 mm to 10 mm in diameter are recommended.[27] We have also used an expandable reamer that allows further debridement in the subchondral region (see Fig. 2C). The bone is then curetted and the tunnel is washed. Radiopaque contrast is injected in the tunnel before grafting to verify that there has been adequate debridement and no intra-articular penetration (see Fig. 2C). Bone grafting is performed with either bone graft substitutes or autograft. Our current preference is to use synthetic material that

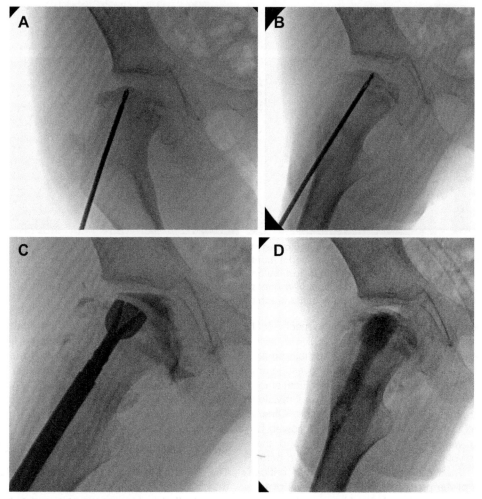

Fig. 2. Technique of core decompression. (*A, B*) The guidewire in the center of the defect. (*C*) Intraoperative image showing the tulip reamer expanding the area of debridement. Note radiopaque dye in the joint to help identify the articular surface. (*D*) After injection of bone graft substitute.

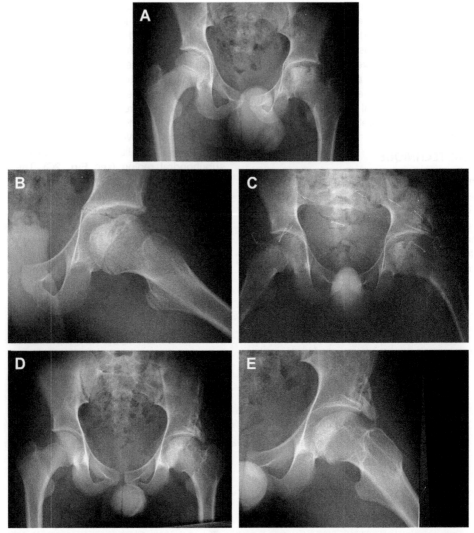

Fig. 3. Core decompression and shelf acetabuloplasty for idiopathic juvenile osteonecrosis. (*A, B*) Anteroposterior and lateral radiographs of a boy 12 years and 4 months old 6 months after onset of symptoms. (*C*) In spica cast following core decompression and shelf acetabuloplasty. (*D, E*) At skeletal maturity, 5 years following core decompression and shelf acetabuloplasty. (*F–I*) Almost equal range of motion. The shelf is larger than desired, but the patient is asymptomatic and engages in athletic activities.

solidifies and provides some early mechanical support before resorption (see **Fig. 2**D).

Several investigators advocate multiple small-diameter drill holes.[22,30,31] These investigators have identified that patients with earlier Ficat stage and smaller lesions (<200°) required less revision surgery than those with larger lesions. Others have performed core decompression followed by grafting with tibia or fibula.[16] They found that patients younger than 30 years of age had better results. They concluded that the most critical portion of the procedure was the removal of the necrotic tissue and packing of bone graft, as the type of strut graft had minimal effect on the procedure. Urbaniak and colleagues[32] used

vascularized fibular grafting and reported 5-year survival rates of 89% for Ficat Stage II hips and 77% for Stage III hips. Regardless of method of bone grafting, authors have reported better outcomes in patients younger than 30 years of age.[16,33]

COMPLICATIONS OF CORE DECOMPRESSION

The literature reports up to 15% complication rate.[15,25,30,31] However, these are reports of adult patients that include pneumonia and pulmonary embolism. The most common complications have been femoral fractures and femoral head blowout.

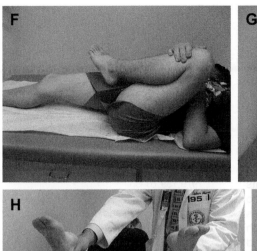
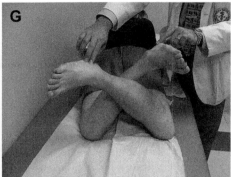
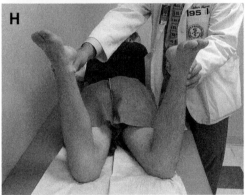
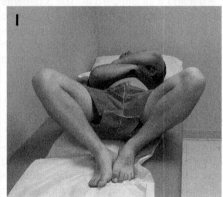

Fig. 3. (*continued*)

A major concern in children is premature growth arrest of the proximal femur. This arrest is expected to occur when large-diameter core decompression is performed. However, the poor prognosis of Perthes disease in the adolescent combined with the limited growth potential of the proximal femur warrants consideration of large-core decompression in older children.

Any drilling across the growth plate leads to bridging bone formation unless metal or other material fills the hole.[50,51] However, central drill holes or involvement of less than 5% of the growth plate have not resulted in growth retardation.[50,51] For this reason, decompression with multiple small drill holes may be considered in younger children or in patients with less severe involvement. The authors have no experience with core decompression in children younger than 10 years of age, and we have no experience with multiple small drilling techniques.

SHELF ACETABULOPLASTY (LABRAL SUPPORT)

Inadequate lateral femoral head coverage has been identified as a risk factor for poor outcomes in adults following core decompression with vascularized fibular grafting.[52] The coverage of the femoral head

is also an important factor for long-term outcome.[53] Saito and colleagues[53] studied the steepness of the upward slope of the lateral acetabular margin and named this the acetabular roof angle. An average acetabular roof angle of $-12.5°$ was positively associated with osteoarthritis at an average follow-up of 18 years. Shelf acetabuloplasty can improve the lateral slope of the acetabulum and provide support for the femoral head. Madan and colleagues[54] evaluated acetabular remodeling potential and recommended acetabular procedures in older children because of reduced capacity for acetabular remodeling with reduced acetabular depth following Perthes disease in older children.

Chiari osteotomy and shelf acetabuloplasty also have provided symptomatic relief and improved function in patients with hinge abduction, coxa magna, or arthrosis following Perthes disease.[55–58] Thus, labral support may be beneficial for older patients who have a more severe prognosis for some residual deformity whether core decompression is performed or not.

AUTHORS' EXPERIENCE

Our preliminary experience with core decompression and shelf acetabuloplasty for older children with idiopathic juvenile osteonecrosis is limited to

6 patients. Average follow-up is 25 months with a range of 12 to 60 months. Only 1 patient has been followed for less than 18 months. Age at time of surgery averaged 12 years with a range of 10.5 to 14.6 years. Two patients were treated in the early fragmentation stage before femoral head collapse. Both of those patients have excellent outcomes, with spherical femoral heads, full range of motion, and no symptoms (**Fig. 3**). The remaining 4 patients had surgery later in the course of disease, including 1 late stage with lateral migration. At follow-up, 1 of these 4 patients is classified as Stulberg II and 3 as Stulberg III. The 3 patients with Stulberg III outcomes have mild limp, but no pain, and they participate in normal daily activities including recreational sports. The 3 patients with Stulberg I or II outcomes are asymptomatic and without limp.

SUMMARY AND RECOMMENDATIONS

The primary goals of treatment of juvenile osteonecrosis are to maintain or promote a round and congruous femoral head that is contained within the acetabulum. Juvenile osteonecrosis does not fare well following observation or treatment by previously reported methods. Surgery is indicated in these patients based on the natural history studies.[1,2,4,7,47] Decompression relieves pain and improves vascularity. Debridement and grafting of the necrotic segment may allow more rapid reconstitution of the femoral head.[1,16,45] The earlier in the course of disease that this is performed, the better the outcomes for preventing femoral head collapse and residual deformity.

Decompression of the femoral head and neck in Perthes disease may be a useful adjunct to current methods of treatment. Several investigators have reported sporadic cases of core decompression in Perthes using large-bore decompression or multiple small drillings.[1,12,13,49] It is our opinion that younger children with early stage disease may benefit from multiple small drillings, but we recommend large-core decompression, debridement, and grafting for Perthes disease in older children with larger lesions and more advanced stages of disease.

REFERENCES

1. Joseph B, Mulpuri K, Varghese G. Perthes' disease in the adolescent. J Bone Joint Surg Br 2001;83(5): 715–20.
2. Ippolito E, Tudisco C, Farsetti P. Long-term prognosis of Legg-Calve-Perthes disease developing during adolescence. J Pediatr Orthop 1985;5(6):652–6.
3. Domzalski ME, Glutting J, Bowen JR, et al. The proximal femoral growth plate in Perthes disease. Clin Orthop Relat Res 2007;458:150–8.
4. Stulberg SD, Cooperman DR, Wallensten R. The natural history of Legg-Calve-Perthes disease. J Bone Joint Surg Am 1981;63(7):1095–108.
5. Ippolito E, Tudisco C, Farsetti P. The long-term prognosis of unilateral Perthes' disease. J Bone Joint Surg Br 1987;69(2):243–50.
6. Thompson GH, Westin GW. Legg-Calve-Perthes disease: results of discontinuing treatment in the early reossification phase. Clin Orthop Relat Res 1979;139:70–80.
7. Mazda K, Penneçot GF, Zeller R, et al. Perthes' disease after the age of twelve years. J Bone Joint Surg Br 1999;81:696–8.
8. Glimcher MJ, Kenzora JE. The biology of osteonecrosis of the human femoral head and its clinical implications. III. Discussion of the etiology and genesis of the pathological sequelae; comments on treatment. Clin Orthop Relat Res 1979;(140):273–312.
9. Hofstaetter JG, Wang J, Yan J, et al. Changes in bone microarchitecture and bone mineral density following experimental osteonecrosis of the hip in rabbits. Cells Tissues Organs 2006;184(3–4):138–47.
10. Ficat R. Idiopathic bone necrosis of the femoral head: early diagnosis and treatment. J Bone Joint Surg Br 1985;67:3–9.
11. Aaron RK, Lennox D, Bunce GE, et al. The conservative treatment of osteonecrosis of the femoral head. A comparison of core decompression and pulsing electromagnetic fields. Clin Orthop Relat Res 1989;(249):209–18.
12. Bozsan EJ. A new treatment of intracapsular fractures of the neck of the femur and Calvé-Legg-Perthes disease. J Bone Joint Surg Am 1932;14:884–7.
13. Ferguson A, Howorth MB. Coxa plana and related conditions of the hip: part II. J Bone Joint Surg 1935;16:789–803.
14. Mont M, Marulanda GA, Seyler TM, et al. Core decompression and nonvascularized bone grafting for the treatment of early stage osteonecrosis of the femoral head. Instr Course Lect 2007;56: 213–20.
15. Mont MA, Carbone JJ, Fairbank AC. Core decompression versus nonoperative management for osteonecrosis of the hip. Clin Orthop Relat Res 1996;(324):169–78.
16. Keizer S, Kock NB, Dijkstra PD, et al. Treatment of avascular necrosis of the hip by a nonvascularized cortical graft. J Bone Joint Surg Br 2006;88(4):460–6.
17. Wells L, Hosalker HS, Crawford EA, et al. Thorough debridement under endoscopic visualization with bone grafting and stabilization for femoral head osteonecrosis in children. J Pediatr Orthop 2009; 29(4):319–26.

18. Govaers K, Meermans G, Bortier H, et al. Endoscopically assisted core decompression in avascular necrosis of the femoral head. Acta Orthop Belg 2009;75(5):631–6.

19. Lee M, Hsieh PH, Chang YH, et al. Elevated intraosseous pressure in the intertrochanteric region is associated with poorer results in osteonecrosis of the femoral head treated by multiple drilling. J Bone Joint Surg Br 2008;90(7):852–7.

20. Iwasaki K. The change in venous circulation of the proximal part of the femur after varus osteotomy in Perthes' disease. Nippon Seikeigeka Gakkai Zasshi 1986;60:237–49.

21. Harris W, Hobson KW. Histological changes in experimentally displaced upper femoral epiphysis in rabbits. J Bone Joint Surg Br 1956;38:914–21.

22. Marker DR, Seyler TM, Ulrich SD, et al. Do modern techniques improve core decompression outcomes for hip osteonecrosis? Clin Orthop Relat Res 2008; 466(5):1093–103.

23. Steinberg ME, Brighton CT, Corces A, et al. Osteonecrosis of the femoral head. Results of core decompression and grafting with and without electrical stimulation. Clin Orthop Relat Res 1989;(249): 199–208.

24. Veillette CJ, Mehdian H, Schemitsch EH, et al. Survivorship analysis and radiographic outcome following tantalum rod insertion for osteonecrosis of the femoral head. J Bone Joint Surg Am 2006; 88(Suppl 3):48–55.

25. Fairbank AC, Bhatia D, Jinnah RH, et al. Long-term results of core decompression for ischaemic necrosis of the femoral head. J Bone Joint Surg Br 1995;77(1): 42–9.

26. Stulberg BN, Davis AW, Bauer TW, et al. Osteonecrosis of the femoral head. A prospective randomized treatment protocol. Clin Orthop Relat Res 1991;(268):140–51.

27. Stulberg BN, Bauer TW, Belhobek GH. Making core decompression work. Clin Orthop Relat Res 1990;(261):186–95.

28. Ficat R, Arlet J. Necrosis of the femoral head. In: Hungerford D, editor. Ischemia and necrosis of bone. Baltimore (MD): Williams & Wilkins; 1980. p. 53–74.

29. Mont M, Marulanda GA, Jones LD, et al. Systematic analysis of classification systems for osteonecrosis of the femoral head. J Bone Joint Surg Am 2006; 88(Suppl 3):16–26.

30. Mont M, Ragland PS, Etienne G. Core decompression of the femoral head for osteonecrosis using percutaneous multiple small-diameter drilling. Clin Orthop Relat Res 2004;429:131–8.

31. Song W, Yoo JJ, Kim YM, et al. Results of multiple drilling compared with those of conventional methods of core decompression. Clin Orthop Relat Res 2006; 454:139–46.

32. Urbaniak JR, Coogan PG, Gunneson EB, et al. Treatment of osteonecrosis of the femoral head with free vascularized fibular grafting. A long-term follow-up study of one hundred and three hips. J Bone Joint Surg Am 1995;77(5).081–94.

33. Boss JH, Misselevich I, Bejar J, et al. Experimentally gained insight-based proposal apropos the treatment of osteonecrosis of the femoral head. Med Hypotheses 2004;62(6):958–65.

34. Mont M, Jones LC, Seyler TM, et al. New treatment approaches for osteonecrosis of the femoral head: an overview. Instr Course Lect 2007;56:197–212.

35. Berend K, Gunneson EE, Urbaniak JR. Free vascularized fibular grafting for the treatment of postcollapse osteonecrosis of the femoral head. J Bone Joint Surg Am 2003;85(6):987–93.

36. Lieberman JR, Conduah A, Urist MR. Treatment of osteonecrosis of the femoral head with core decompression and human bone morphogenetic protein. Clin Orthop Relat Res 2004;(429):139–45.

37. Chang T, Tang K, Tao X, et al. Treatment of early avascular necrosis of femoral head by core decompression combined with autologous bone marrow mesenchymal stem cells transplantation. Zhongguo Xiu Fu Chong Jian Wai Ke Za Zhi 2010;24(6):739–43 [in Chinese].

38. Dean G, Kime RC, Fitch RD, et al. Treatment of osteonecrosis in the hip of pediatric patients by free vascularized fibular graft. Clin Orthop Relat Res 2001;386:106–13.

39. Steinberg ME, Bands RE, Parry S, et al. Does lesion size affect the outcome in avascular necrosis? Clin Orthop Relat Res 1999;(367):262–71.

40. Steinberg ME, Larcom PG, Strafford B, et al. Core decompression with bone grafting for osteonecrosis of the femoral head. Clin Orthop Relat Res 2001;(386):71–8.

41. Mont MA, Zywiel MG, Marker DR, et al. The natural history of untreated asymptomatic osteonecrosis of the femoral head: a systematic literature review. J Bone Joint Surg Am 2010;92(12):2165–70.

42. Chan TW, Dalinka MK, Steinberg ME, et al. MRI appearance of femoral head osteonecrosis following core decompression and bone grafting. Skeletal Radiol 1991;20(2):103–7.

43. Koo KH, Kim R. Quantifying the extent of osteonecrosis of the femoral head. A new method using MRI. J Bone Joint Surg Br 1995;77(6):875–80.

44. Ha YC, Jung WH, Kim JR, et al. Prediction of collapse in femoral head osteonecrosis: a modified Kerboul method with use of magnetic resonance images. J Bone Joint Surg Am 2006;88(Suppl 3): 35–40.

45. Mont MA, Jones LC, Pacheco I, et al. Radiographic predictors of outcome of core decompression for hips with osteonecrosis stage III. Clin Orthop Relat Res 1998;(354):159–68.

46. Mont MA, Ragland PS, Parvizi J. Surgical treatment of osteonecrosis of the hip. Instr Course Lect 2006; 55:167–72.

47. Daly K, Bruce C, Catterall A. Lateral shelf acetabuloplasty in Perthes' disease. A review of the end of growth. J Bone Joint Surg Br 1999;81(3):380–4.

48. Yoo WJ, Choi IH, Cho TJ, et al. Shelf acetabuloplasty for children with Perthes' disease and reducible subluxation of the hip: prognostic factors related to hip remodelling. J Bone Joint Surg Br 2009;91(10): 1383–7.

49. Baksi D. Palliative operations for painful old Perthes' disease. Int Orthop 1995;19:46–50.

50. Garces L, Mucica-Garay I, Coviella NL, et al. Growth-plate modifications after drilling. J Pediatr Orthop 1994;14:225–8.

51. Janarv PM, Wikstrom B, Hirsch G. The influence of transphyseal drilling and tendon grafting on bone growth: an experimental study in the rabbit. J Pediatr Orthop 1998;18(2):149–54.

52. Roush TF, Olson SA, Pietrobon R, et al. Influence of acetabular coverage on hip survival after free vascularized fibular grafting for femoral head osteonecrosis. J Bone Joint Surg Am 2006;88(10):2152–8.

53. Saito S, Takoaka K, Ono K, et al. Residual deformities related to arthrotic change after Perthes' disease. A long-term follow-up of fifty-one cases. Arch Orthop Trauma Surg 1985;104(1):7–14.

54. Madan S, Fernandes J, Taylor JF. Radiological remodeling of the acetabulum in Perthes' disease. Acta Orthop Belg 2003;69(5):412–20.

55. Koyama K, Higuchi F, Inoue A. Modified Chiari osteotomy for arthrosis after Perthes' disease. Acta Orthop Scand 1998;69:129–32.

56. Freeman R, Wainwright AM, Theologis TN, et al. The outcome of patients with hinge abduction in severe Perthes' disease treated by shelf acetabuloplasty. J Pediatr Orthop 2008;28:619–25.

57. Schepers A, von Bormann PF, Craig JJ. Coxa magna in Perthes' disease: treatment by Chiari pelvic osteotomy. J Bone Joint Surg Br 1978; 60:297.

58. Klisic P. Treatment of Perthes' disease in older children. J Bone Joint Surg Br 1983;65:419–27.

Consensus Statements on the Management of Perthes Disease

Consensus Statement	Agree	Agree with Minor Change	Agree/Disagree in Part	Disagree
Goals of Treatment of Legg-Calvé-Perthes Disease				
1. The primary long-term goal of treatment of Legg-Calvé-Perthes disease is to try to prevent secondary degenerative arthritis of the hip in adult life by achieving the short-term goal cited next (2)	GT, I-HC, TH, GH, JH-S, HK, DE, DGL, CP, BJ			
2. The primary short-term goal of treatment of Legg-Calvé-Perthes disease is to try to ensure that when the disease is completely healed the femoral head is spherical, and minimally enlarged (ie, prevent the femoral head from getting deformed)	GT, I-HC, TH, GH, HK, DGL, CP, BJ	JH-S, DE		
TREATMENT OF LEGG-CALVÉ-PERTHES DISEASE: TIME FRAMES				
3. The treatment of Legg-Calvé-Perthes disease needs to be divided into 3 distinct time frames: a. *Early in the course of the disease*: this first and most vital frame is from the onset of the disease to the early fragmentation stage b. *Late in the course of the disease*: this second time frame is from the late fragmentation stage to full reossification of the femoral head (complete healing) c. *After complete healing*: the third time frame is after the disease has healed and residual sequelae are present The aims of treatment will necessarily vary in each of these 3 time frames. The options and the strategies of treatment will also vary in each of these 3 time frames	GT, I-HC, TH, GH, JH-S, HK, DGL, CP, BJ		DE	
TREATMENT EARLY IN THE COURSE OF THE DISEASE				
4. The goal of treatment early in the course of the disease is to retain the normal shape of the femoral head by: a. Identifying patients at risk for a poor outcome as soon as possible b. Containing the femoral head as early as possible in patients at risk of a poor outcome	GT, I-HC, GH, JH-S, CP, BJ	TH, DE	HK, DGL	
5. Containment may be achieved by nonoperative or operative means and surgical options include femoral and /or pelvic surgery	GT, I-HC, TH, GH, JH-S, HK, DGL, CP, BJ	DE		

(continued on next page)

Orthop Clin N Am 42 (2011) 437–440
doi:10.1016/j.ocl.2011.05.001
0030-5898/11/$ – see front matter © 2011 Elsevier Inc. All rights reserved.

Consensus Statement	Agree	Agree with Minor Change	Agree/Disagree in Part	Disagree
6. Containment may or may not be combined with weight relief	I-HC, TH, GH, JH-S, HK, DGL, CP, BJ	DE		GT
7. In order for containment to be successful, it should be achieved before the late stage of fragmentation	GT, I-HC, TH, GH, JH-S, HK, DGL, CP, BJ		DE	
8. Containment should be maintained until the late reconstitution (reossification) stage	GT, I-HC, TH, GH, JH-S, HK, DGL, CP, BJ	DE		
9. The decision to consider containment treatment early in the course of the disease is primarily governed by the age of onset of the disease with patients divided into 4 age groups. (The chronologic age is used in most centers in the decision making as skeletal age atlases are not available for several ethnic populations and because there is a lack of natural history data based on skeletal age)	GT, I-HC, TH, GH, JH-S, DGL, CP, BJ	HK		DE
10. Children less than 5 years of age at the onset of the disease: treatment is seldom needed regardless of severity of involvement of the femoral head. (However, if femoral head extrusion occurs treatment will be needed)	GT, GH, JH-S, DGL, CP, BJ	I-HC, TH, DE, HK		
11. Children 5 years or older but less than 8 years of age at onset of the disease: a. Early containment is indicated if it is possible to determine that more than half the femoral epiphysis is necrotic b. Early determination cannot be made in most patients. These patients should be monitored with periodic (~4-monthly) radiographs to detect early extrusion of the femoral head c. Containment treatment should be considered as soon as extrusion of the femoral head is detected (provided the disease has not progressed into the late stage of fragmentation) d. Extrusion is determined by a break in the Shenton line or the Reimer migration index >20% e. No containment is need in this age group when extrusion does not occur	GT, GH, JH-S, CP, BJ	I-HC, TH, DE	HK, DGL	
12. Children 8 years or older but less than 12 years of age at onset of the disease: a. Should be treated by containment as soon as the disease is diagnosed regardless of the extent of necrosis. Containment should be initiated before the fragmentation stage and before extrusion whenever possible b. Alternative methods should be considered when the patient presents in the late stage of fragmentation	GT, I-HC, GH, JH-S, CP, BJ	TH, HK, DE		DGL

(continued on next page)

Consensus Statement	Agree	Agree with Minor Change	Agree/ Disagree in Part	Disagree
13. Children 12 years of age or older at the onset of the disease: containment should NOT be considered in these adolescents as it does not work. Treatment considerations should be similar to treatment of adults with osteonecrosis	GT, I-HC, GH, CP, BJ	TH, JH-S, DE, HK, DGL		
TREATMENT LATE IN THE COURSE OF THE DISEASE				
14. The goal of treatment of Legg-Calvé-Perthes late in the course of the disease is to attempt to minimize the extent of deformation of the femoral head that has already developed from extrusion	GT, I-HC, TH, GH, HK, DE, DGL, CP, BJ			
15. The treatment in the late fragmentation stage may be remedial or salvage depending on the deformity of the femoral head or the presence of hinge abduction. In children who have hinge abduction the goal of treatment is to correct hinge abduction and facilitate some remodeling of the femoral head	GT, I-HC, TH, GH, JH-S, HK, DGL, CP, BJ		DE	
16. Containment may be considered if the femoral head can be contained without hinge abduction. (In these late cases, the prognosis for obtaining a spherical femoral head is guarded)	GT, I-HC, TH, GH, JH-S, HK, DGL, CP, BJ	DE		
17. If hinge abduction is present, containment is unlikely to improve the femoral head shape. A valgus femoral osteotomy is a reliable choice to improve motion and reduce pain	GT, I-HC, GH, JH-S, CP, BJ	TH, DE	HK, DGL	
TREATMENT AFTER HEALING OF THE DISEASE				
18. The goals of treatment of adolescents or young adults with healed Legg-Calvé-Perthes disease and deformity of the femoral head is to improve function, relive pain, and delay the onset of secondary degenerative arthritis	GT, I-HC TH, GH, JH-S, HK, DE, DGL, CP, BJ			
19. The treatment approach depends on the specific cause of pain, dysfunction, or deformity	GT, I-HC, TH, GH, JH-S, HK, DE, DGL, CP, BJ			
20. If the femoral head is spherical or ovoid and there is coxa brevis with a Trendelenburg gait, consider trochanteric advancement with or without lengthening the femoral neck	GT, I-HC, TH, GH, JH-S, HK, DGL, CP, BJ	DE		
21. If there is pain on account of femoro-acetabular impingement consider repairing the labral pathology and/or correcting impingement	GT, I-HC, TH, JH-S, DE, DGL, CP, BJ		HK	
22. A deficient acetabular roof may require labral support or pelvic osteotomy with or without realignment of the proximal femur	GT, I-HC, TH, GH, JH-S, DE, DGL, CP, BJ		HK	

(continued on next page)

Consensus Statement	Agree	Agree with Minor Change	Agree/ Disagree in Part	Disagree
23. Symptoms caused by osteochondritis dessicans can sometimes be relieved by removing the loose fragment	GT, I-HC, TH, GH, JH-S, H, DGL, CP, BJ	DE		
24. The role of reshaping a grossly deformed femoral head is uncertain although in a few selected cases of moderate deformity, it may be of benefit	GT, I-HC, TH, GH, JH-S, DE, CP, BJ		HK, DGL	
25. When the articular surface is severely damaged salvage procedures such a total hip replacement should be considered	GT, I-HC, TH, GH, JH-S, DGL, CP, BJ	HK, DE		

Keys: BJ, Benjamin Joseph; CP, Charles Price; DE, Deborah Eastwood; DGL, David G Little; GH, Gamal Hosny; GT, George Thompson; HK, Harry Kim; I-HC, In-Ho Choi; JH-S, Jose Herrara-Soto; TH, Tony Herring.

Benjamin Joseph, MS Orth, MCh Orth
Kasturba Medical College
Manipal 576 104
Karnataka State, India

Charles T. Price, MD
Arnold Palmer Hospital for Children
Specialty Practices Pediatric Orthopaedics
83 West Columbia Street
Orlando, FL 32806, USA

E-mail addresses:
bjosephortho@yahoo.co.in (B. Joseph)
charles.price@orlandohealth.com (C.T. Price)

Index

Note: Page numbers of article titles are in **boldface** type.

Orthop Clin N Am 42 (2011) 441–445
doi:10.1016/S0030-5898(11)00051-4
0030-5898/11/$ – see front matter © 2011 Elsevier Inc. All rights reserved.

orthopedic.theclinics.com

Moving?

Make sure your subscription moves with you!

To notify us of your new address, find your **Clinics Account Number** (located on your mailing label above your name), and contact customer service at:

Email: journalscustomerservice-usa@elsevier.com

800-654-2452 (subscribers in the U.S. & Canada)
314-447-8871 (subscribers outside of the U.S. & Canada)

Fax number: 314-447-8029

Elsevier Health Sciences Division
Subscription Customer Service
3251 Riverport Lane
Maryland Heights, MO 63043

*To ensure uninterrupted delivery of your subscription, please notify us at least 4 weeks in advance of move.

Printed and bound by CPI Group (UK) Ltd, Croydon, CR0 4YY

03/10/2024

01040350-0013